Diaries of a
Mad Nurse

Revealing
The True Culprits of Disease

Marty A. Robins

DEDICATION

This book is dedicated to all people
who have suffered and are suffering needlessly.

A NOTE TO READERS

The brand name products mentioned in this book are registered trademarks. The companies that own these trademarks and make these products do not endorse, recommend, or accept any liability for any use of their products other than those uses indicated on the package labels or in current company brochures. At no time, should this book be regarded as a substitute for professional medical treatment. This book contains opinions and ideas of its author. The author has compiled the information contained within from a variety of sources. Neither the author, publisher, manufacturers, nor distributors assume any legal responsibility for any problems arising from its suggestions or experimentation with the methods described herein.

CONTENTS

ACKNOWLEDGMENTS

To the many thousands of people who I have had the honor of taking care of, I thank you. It is through the history of your lives that I have been encouraged to write about such a controversial issue as healthcare. Your insights, as well as your lack of insights into this problem are what this book will be based upon.

To my family and friends: I thank you for your support and encouragement during the writing of this book. It was this precious time away from all, which gave me the ability to answer the many questions within.

To Ted: Without your impeccable insight into health, I would never have looked at this issue in its entirety.

To Debbie and Sonja: I thank you for your shared talents and your editorial expertise in the completion of this book.

To Tracy: Without the inspirational guidance of your Right Living Program, I would have never been able to express the principles that are so necessary for these needed changes in our lives.

To the medical profession: I thank you for giving me a career of many years, where I have learned right from wrong.

And to God, I thank you for the ability to believe.

INTRODUCTION

It is for the sake of humanity that I have written this book.

Diaries of a Mad Nurse is based on my personal journals, collected over many years of caring for thousands of people and the hard-learned and often heartbreaking lessons of a medical professional. During my career, a dream began to take root. I wanted to find a way to help people become healthier, while promoting a better level of personal awareness. My dream was not only to write a book on health, but to write a book that would educate and inspire every individual to attain more self-reliance when it comes to managing his or her own care.

Today, America's healthcare system is in a crisis. Not only is it compromised and over-utilized, but it is most of all, over spent. As we examine this dilemma, we must ask ourselves one very important question. *Are the American people truly receiving a standard of healthcare that is beneficial to all?*

Yes, people are living longer. However, are they actually living a life that gives them a level of greater well-being? We need only to look to the elderly, who arrive at our hospitals from nursing homes and assisted living facilities suffering from contractures, dementia, depression, and other debilitating diseases to see that this is not always the case.

Within this book, one will often see the word *quality*. This simple word is one I will focus on to address the reasons why *health* care has lost its meaning for so many. Today, we are dealing with quantity and not always quality, and this is why we are seeing a decline of the healthcare industry in this country. Through my experiences and personal observations of some of these absurdities of this modern healthcare system, I came to realize that this book desperately needed to be written.

Surely, healthcare has many factors and reasons to why it has created its many problems. Yet, before we can ever understand the need for a new standard of healthcare that will be successful, it is imperative that we analyze in depth the existing difficulties with the current system. It will be through this acknowledgement and examination of what is wrong with healthcare today, that we will ultimately discover what is necessary to create a better healthcare for tomorrow.

As we all know, there are too many people without healthcare: fifty million people and growing as I write this. However, before we can even approach this problem, we must answer yet another serious question. *Is it our responsibility to support the people who are exploiting our healthcare system?* This includes the American government, insurance companies, major pharmaceutical companies, special interest groups, illegal immigrants, and consumers themselves.

Within these pages, I will reflect upon many of the lifestyle choices of individuals I have encountered during my career, where their choices have led them, and what they really need to do in order to learn how to obtain optimal health. I will examine not only the specific actions and beliefs of these individuals, but the actions and beliefs of many others. These personal diaries will present a clearer perspective to the pathways of improving one's health by giving you, the consumer, the necessary information to develop a more precise and rational way of caring for yourself.

What I will show is how to be less dependent on our current healthcare system while learning to be more independent in your healthcare choices. I will also examine the fundamentals of disease from a very different aspect and offer real world, practical solutions to some of the problems caused by chronic diseases. My ultimate goal is to teach people that the path to good health begins with you, and I want very much to help you get there.

CHAPTER 1

LET'S LOOK AT THE REAL PROBLEM

Whether with healthcare or on a personal level, the real problems in this world today stem from greed and lack of accountability. Rich or poor, we all want more. How sad it is that most of us focus on what we want, rather than what we truly need. While we often deny what is going on inside ourselves, we remain preoccupied with what is occurring only on the outside. For many, this is simply just an issue of increasing one's self-awareness.

For the most part, we are no longer a nation of positive thinking people, but rather we have become a society that lives in fear and negativity. To recognize this fact, we need only to turn on our televisions or computers to see the latest news. There we will observe killings, mortgage and credit card default, foreclosures, oil spills, earthquakes, tsunamis, and other catastrophes. All of these life occurrences have helped bring us to an unacceptable level of chaos and stress within ourselves.

With much of this chaos being felt in the financial world, people are finally taking a closer look at where they are and where they need to be. This recession has most of us analyzing our financial problems and setting new priorities. Yet, for some people, they continue to be oblivious to these facts. They continue to spend their money on superfluous materialism and meaningless objects. Many have just ignored the necessity of saving for this rainy day. We need only to look at the number of households that are falling apart due to financial problems. Clearly, some people have not yet learned what it takes to survive in these times of financial and emotional woes.

As a nation, we have also had to deal with a younger generation who believes that they deserve everything without ever being required to work for it. Of course, there are exceptions to this finding, but many young adults are now facing this rude yet valid awakening. Should we not all question the importance of these situations and ask ourselves, "Where are we, as individuals, actually going?"

As work, or lack of work, carries us from day to day, we must ask ourselves how happy and contented we are when we reflect on our lives. Are we living in peace, tranquility and joy, or are we lost in a state of flux and denial? Are our lives safe, and do we actually have *control* over what we wish for? I call this an *inevitable downfall of self.*

In these difficult times, we must also address some other relevant questions: Is a paycheck the only satisfaction we are receiving from our labors? Are we living the life we dreamed about? Are we utilizing the very special talents we have been given? Do we realize how truly unique and special we all are? Perhaps most important, we need to ask ourselves if these are the true realities of our lives.

Of course, there are many people who do maintain their status quo and appear to be content, but for many others, life has presented itself with excruciating, if not insurmountable, obstacles. Only observe the many people who work and work and work. These *workaholics* insist they need to work long hours for their financial security. For many this is true, yet for others, the main reason they work so compulsively hard and keep such busy lifestyles is to avoid having to deal with themselves. They cannot acknowledge their emotional emptiness, nor do they ever question how they got to where they are. Their inability to look deeply within themselves, and be aware of their inner problems, only adds to their refusal to create self-awareness or even share intimacy with others. Consider the rising divorce statistics, increasing depression and suicide rates. These issues are occurring in the lives of many, which are a result of a lifetime of avoidance of oneself and the reality of their existing situations.

You may be asking yourself how this relates to your health. I believe there is a very profound correlation. When a human being denies their true authentic self, they deny who they truly are. With this loss of authenticity of self, as well as all of the other stresses in this world today, a human being can and will enter into a place filled with many levels and forms of illness.

When human beings find themselves in stressful situations, they quite often discover they have less control over their lives. Faced with this lack of control, many find they do not feel perfectly safe. As challenges multiply, consciously and unconsciously, they can take people to a place where their bodies will turn against them and they will begin to see a variety of effects that manifest as illnesses. These circumstances bring about increased potential for disease and people must realize that these experiences can and will eventually take hold of their lives. Although, diseases can certainly present themselves in many ways, we must educate ourselves to look at illness beyond what we have been taught. What we need to acknowledge correctly is that <u>*our minds and emotions definitely affect the health of our bodies.*</u>

Today's standard practice is to look at illness usually on a physical level. However, is it possible that the medical profession as a whole is ignoring an important psychological implication to disease? I believe that they are. We must remember that we are not only physical beings; we are emotional beings as well. Because of this, I believe it is not heart disease, stroke, or cancers that are the leading causes of death, but instead they are the result of one's lack of self-awareness and insight. I will show how *one's toxic emotional input into one's self* becomes a primary and leading cause and culprit of the many diseases that currently exist.

As a nation, we can no longer jump into solutions that have failed us in the past. We need to learn the actual and fundamental reasons for illnesses so that we can create a more humane and positive way to obtain a quality of health that will be beneficial to all. When this is understood, we will not only attain personal accountability and mindfulness for our health, but we will become advocates for ourselves as well as for others.

DIARIES OF A MAD NURSE

CHAPTER 2

LET'S LOOK AT ILLNESS

I have found that when people are seeking care from practitioners, they have some idea of why they are ill. They present themselves with a symptom or a complaint that profoundly states "Help me." This statement belies the underlying fact that there is much more here than what the patient is saying. For this reason, we shall now examine illness from a very different point of view.

I believe it is often a fundamental lack of self-understanding that allows many of us to fall into these states of illness. Granted, there are various circumstances, such as congenital abnormalities, structural problems, and accidents, which speak for themselves. Yet, what about the illnesses that do not have such obvious reasons for why someone is ill?

As individuals, we most certainly have increased demands placed on us daily. These demands can be either positive or negative. Since positive influences usually have positive effects on our bodies, we will concentrate solely on the effects of these negative influences. I will describe how certain self-generated negative input can become one of the main reasons why so many people are ill. We will learn not only how to improve and treat illnesses differently, but how we can also achieve a healthier outcome in our lives.

As we all know, a human being consists of a body, a mind, and for some people a soul. By not understanding this important body, mind, soul interconnectedness, much of healthcare has fallen short. We find that traditional medicine believes often that disease is predominantly of the body, not of the mind. Because of this belief, we will now reveal how important this mind-body-soul connection is, learn exactly what can affect it, and how those effects can cause illness.

When someone complains of things like a headache, backache, or stomach pain, he is a patient with a physical ailment. When someone overdoses, has an anxiety/panic attack, or confesses suicidal thoughts, he is classified as a patient with an emotional problem. The medical community acknowledges this. However, what if our illnesses are what I call a check and balance system, requiring us to look deeper to find what is actually causing these illnesses? Could it be that what has affected us emotionally in the past, or even the present be the true reason and culprit for why we are sick today?

To answer this question more fully, let us begin by saying that *toxic emotions can be underestimated, and if not treated, they will become harmful to our bodies.* While the effects of theses emotions will be investigated, solutions to these emotional problems will also be discussed as we consider the implications of this very significant statement.

THE EMOTION OF ANGER:

Experiencing this emotion is a sign that something is wrong. This emotion will get others' attention as well as our own. It lets us know when we are being violated, and when someone or something is harming us. It is often a reaction to unfair circumstances. Although we are often taught that anger is wrong and that we must control it, we must also realize it can be right. Anger can be protective. Only think of a mother screaming at her child who is running into the path of an oncoming car. This example of anger protects her child from harm. Her anger has become a tool to keep her child safe. This is called *hot anger* and in many circumstances can be good for an individual. Hot anger allows our stress to focus outwardly.

Cold anger, on the other hand, focuses inward. It can injure not only the body, but also the mind and soul. When, we keep this emotion in our bodies, it will produce an environment where illness can, and does, begin. This starts a cycle of checks and balances, which will bury this anger and cause unresolved emotions to stay within our bodies. Soon, we begin to generate a variety of symptoms, which will eventually lead to disease. We start to have backaches, headaches, stomachaches, diarrhea, constipation, cancer, fibromyalgia, lupus, and the list goes on.

Anger, especially repressed anger, has been shown to hurt the liver, gall bladder, heart, and other organs and muscles of the body. It affects the eyes, blood sugar, and blood pressure. An antidote for this emotion is to develop compassion for yourself, as well as, for others.

Traditional medicine does not have all the answers to illness, but what really infuriates me is the insistence on treating a patient without ever con-sidering other potential reasons for why a patient becomes ill. While doctors continue to treat the pain and symptoms, rarely do they think of the patient's emotional thoughts and life events that may have caused many of these illnesses. Has the patient ever been examined for these negative emotions that lie within?

THE EMOTION OF GRIEF:

This is the emotion of intense suffering caused by loss. It can be the loss of someone or something. It is sorrow. The emotion of grief is a very powerful one. We often see many people who are grieving develop cancer and other debilitating diseases, when confronted with this emotion.

When in grief, one always needs to remember to drink plenty of water. In this highly emotional state, the water balance of one's body is usually off. Since water is essential to sustain health, when suffering from grief, one often under-consumes this important component that is so necessary for the flow of life. Only when grieving has taken its course, does a person once again begin to have a life filled with happiness and pleasure.

As a nurse, I have too often seen patients and their families having difficulties dealing with their grief. For this reason, I would now like to reflect on the cases of two well-known celebrities, and show exactly how their grief played a significant role in their deaths.

The first case is the life of Dana Reeves, wife of movie star Christopher Reeves. How did this woman who never smoked develop lung cancer? Yes, it could be said that it was the result of second hand smoke or other environmental toxins. However, could her cancer possibly have come from all the stress during her extreme level of emotional turmoil she sustained for over nine years? Was the ultimate reason for her illness and eventual death a result of her grief and sorrow? Look even deeper and consider why the area involved was her lungs. Was not the breath of her life and her soul taken from her when her husband died? Are not the heart and lungs connected?

Another case history is the life of Michael Jackson. The final diagnosis was presumably accidental overdose. But consider his underlying emotions of isolation, fear, *grief,* sorrow, anger and depression during his life. Were not all of these emotions present in this man? Were not these the initial culprits that led to why he ultimately became dependent on drugs and eventually caused him to lose his life?

When examining the emotion of grief, it has been found to cause damage to the lungs, large intestines, and skin. It impairs one's oxygen metabolism and can be destructive to the thymus and pituitary glands. These two organs affect your immune system, and can often alter your blood pressure and metabolism. One antidote for this emotion is to find the courage to bring joy and laughter back into your life.

THE EMOTION OF SYMPATHY:

Sympathy is the act or capacity for sharing the same feelings as someone else, often equated with *compassion* or *empathy*. Although at times, it is a wonderful emotion to have, we must keep in mind that it can also be detrimental to a person. Sympathy can harm the stomach and can also decrease your blood sugar. Often, I have seen many people who are very sympathetic with others, yet show very little sympathy to themselves. Thus, an antidote for this emotion is to learn how to get angry or mad enough to eventually get up and get going with your own life. Begin to realize it is the present life you need to live in, and do not remain in mourning for the past.

THE EMOTION OF FEAR:

Fear is an unpleasant and often strong emotion caused by the awareness or anticipation of danger. Many people can relate to this emotion when it is called anxiety. It can damage the adrenals, the kidneys and can cause digestive disturbances. Fear often will cause avoidance of others and self that will eventually result in isolation and withdrawal. An antidote for this emotion is to learn to have reverence for one's self as well as for others. This will most assuredly help in many of these frightful situations.

Though only a few emotions have been discussed here, many people who are suffering with illness need to look deeply within themselves for the answers. This profound finding about illness needs much more personal and professional introspection and recognition. With this being said, let us now look at some other emotional issues that trigger the development of disease. These are the problems of *abuse* and *abandonment*. We often find these powerful emotions in the lives of people who are ill. They are of significant importance when it comes to understanding the many causes for disease.

THE ISSUE OF ABUSE:

Abuse is defined as ill treatment, an instance of injustice, or the use of something other than the purpose for which it was intended. In order to fully comprehend the impact of this statement on a person's health, one needs to examine one's own life for any misuse or mistreatment of self in order to understand what actually has occurred.

When it comes to abuse, people must educate themselves. One must realize that the words and actions of others can and will do harm to us if presented in a negative way. One must understand the significant role that these physical and emotional scars of abuse can make to our minds, and realize how any form of this kind of mistreatment can affect our bodies.

Abuse can present itself in many ways and occur at any time in our lives. These abuses can be physical, sexual, spiritual, financial, emotional or verbal. Since they are all of meaningful importance, each one will be examined so that we can more fully understand how they can truly affect a person's life, and even the lives of their entire families.

PHYSICAL ABUSE

When it comes to physical abuse, many people think only of the obvious physical attacks on an individual. However, there is much more than overt physical signs. The physical scars are miniscule in comparison to the emotional ramifications of this kind of mistreatment. Witness the lack of self worth, lack of self-esteem, and especially the significant lack of self-love when it comes to the victim. The physical as well as the emotional scars give us the true picture of what physical abuse actually is.

To elaborate on this topic of physical abuse, one needs only to look at underprivileged areas in this world, where we see children raising children, or orphanages where little care or attention is provided for so many in need. Here, one becomes aware of the real meaning of physical deprivation and abuse. Not only are these children not allowed to be children, they are not *nourished* in the ways children need to be. In most instances, these children are deprived of the physical touch necessary for emotional nurturing to take place. Often they are neglected, abused, and even misused. Early death rates and developmental problems in these children are very often seen.

Our elderly population is a living testimony to this fact that all people need to be acknowledged and touched in positive ways. If not, many ultimately give up on life due to increased isolation, loss of partners, loss of occupations, and the realities of growing old. Today, statistics show the elderly have one of the highest rates of suicide. Studies have also shown that people need to be touched at least twelve times a day in order to have a good sense of self. To this, we must all ask ourselves, "If we are not victims to this sort of abuse?"

Without human contact, many people will find themselves with less of a solid foundation in their lives. It is in this *lack* of physical contact where one becomes abused or abusive. Only consider how the technology of today has limited and changed the factor of this needed human connection.

SEXUAL ABUSE

Sexual abuse takes many forms. It has reached epidemic levels in our society. Types of sexual abuse include rape, unwanted fondling, inappropriate gestures, or even forced subservience to sex. There is also the issue of sex being used for the sake of recreation rather than the purpose of intimacy and growth. We must realize how this kind of abuse can affect the health of its victims and their families. Today, how underestimated this issue of sexual abuse can be.

FINANCIAL ABUSE

Financial abuse takes value and power away from an individual. It can lead a person to a place where they do not feel safe or in control of their lives. A question to be asked when one abuses their finances is, "Do I feel more vulnerable and more helpless when I am without?" Many people's fears and sorrows are vividly exhibited here when this abuse occurs. An example of this is the person who loses their family, home, friends, and career as a result of gambling.

SPIRITUAL ABUSE

Spiritual abuse damages our relationship with God, as well as the essence of our own existence. An example of this is the parent who blames God for taking a child away, or the patient who blames God for an illness. Their own statements of whom to blame are reflective of their own beliefs, or rather lack of beliefs.

VERBAL and EMOTIONAL ABUSE

Not only can the power of the tongue kill one's spirit, it most definitely damages one's essence. We must remember, words were created to foster love and kindness, not to foster pain and untruths. Words were created to empower, not to destroy. How many people can examine their words for what they are worth? How many people can look at what they have suffered and realize that it no longer needs to be? This lack of truth used in verbally abusive situations affects how one treats themselves and others. It creates what I call, "holes in people's souls." We must all look inwardly when dealing with these issues of verbal and emotional abuses.

THE ISSUE OF ABANDONMENT:

Abandonment means to leave or forsake another. When looking at abandonment, we must realize that as others may abandon us, we can also abandon ourselves. Although many say they have never been abandoned, I do not agree. If one is from a single parent family, then they were abandoned. If one grew up with both parents who were not emotionally or physically present, they were abandoned. If any of the abuses mentioned previously were also present, one was not only abused, but they were also abandoned. If a child is not nurtured, they were abandoned. If one's dreams and desires were not supported, they were abandoned. If one gave love and received no love in return, once again, they were abandoned.

Often, this list is very long. If we were to look again at the number of people who actually suffer from abandonment issues, the findings would be startling. If a child grows up without necessary nourishment of self, thet will be an individual who is deprived and dependent. Through this deprivation and dependency, we will see how the issues of abandonment eventually lead to a cause and effect in the development of illness.

When a human being does not believe in self, they will remain dependent on others to complete themselves. When a person becomes ill, this is exactly what takes place. Patients will often become too dependent on a healthcare system to give them the answers and treatments for most of their physical and emotional symptoms. They look outside themselves rather than within. They tend to exclude themselves rather than ask the important question of why and how they have become sick. They continue to avoid and neglect what has gone on in the past and what is going on presently which has brought them to their existing problems and illnesses. They do not acknowledge how their emotions, abuses, or abandonments factor into their disease. Often they suffer from the inability to be mindful.

I have often heard the question, "Why do women live longer than men?" Since women are considered more emotional than men, this is one reason why women live longer. When one releases their emotions in a healthy way, such as crying or discussing their emotions, they free themselves from the physical damages that these suppressed emotions can cause. When patients become more aware of this impact that these issues can have on their health, only then can they finally begin to address the true origins of many of their own illnesses. Thus, it is of the utmost importance to always remain mindful.

Let us now consider some of these diseases that

have taken our independence and power away from us. What we will find is that many of these diseases are self-created. Through acknowledgement and accountability, we are now about to learn how to look at the state of our health and how to question ourselves when it comes to our healthcare choices.

DIARIES OF A MAD NURSE

CHAPTER 3

LET'S LOOK AT SOME DISEASES

OBESITY:

This is an illness of energy balance. More calories in than out plus a lack of physical exercise have been said to be the main causes why people are overweight or obese. Yet, we know that anyone who is overweight has lots of company. The American obesity rates are the highest in the world. Sixty-three percent of adults are categorized as overweight with one third being clinically obese. As of 2012, one in three children were obese or overweight. For the year 2011, seventeen percent of children two to nineteen years of age were obese. This is approximately twelve and a half million children. With these statistics, we must acknowledge that this is one of the fastest growing diseases in America today. It has many factors, such as genetics, family history, age, cultural background, and certain pre-existing conditions. Illnesses such as thyroid and other hormonal disorders have also played their part with this disease. We must not forget that drugs like steroids and antidepressants likewise play a role in this weight dilemma. Although these findings are statistically proven, the most significant precursors to this disease are the factors of environment and lifestyle that we choose. The couch potato society and the fast food mentality need to be looked at as contributing factors to our expanding waistlines.

To those of you who are considered obese, some thirty percent of Americans, I say, "Take off your clothes and look at yourself in the mirror. Are you truly happy with what you see?" If you can honestly say you are, then you are where you need to be.

However, if you are not happy with what you observe, the next question is, *Why do you feel so unimportant that you do not need to take care of your own health and well being?*

Unfortunately, society today puts an enormous emphasis on how and what we should look like. If one is a healthy individual, this should not matter. But the question still remains... why do so many people choose to push society away? Is it the constant attention that they seek, and receive, from the ups and downs of losing weight or is it the sheer addiction to food? As with all problems or addictions, we must realize the message it often sends is, "I do not deserve."

DIABETES:

If one suffers from being overweight or obese, they will probably develop this disease. This disease is not only linked to genetics, lifestyle, and diet also, but it has been linked to many other diseases increasing its high mortality rates. Often, I see people taking their oral hypoglycemic medications or insulin injections only to find out that they are continuing their unhealthy compulsive ways of eating and drinking. I find their lack of control perplexing. Now do not get me wrong, of course, many times people follow a decent diet, exercise regularly, and adhere to a proper diabetic regimen. However, too often, I will see many patients who just cannot accept their disease. These people remain overweight suffering from neuropathy, lack of energy, and other serious complications. Even when they pop that pill or take that injection, most often, they are the ones who choose to stay obese, remain sedentary, and continue their out-of-control lives. In so many words, they are the ones who continue their own abuse.

Frequently, we hear from diabetics that they have

a family history of this disease. They say the main reason they have this disease is because their mother, father, brother, or sister had it. However, do they realize that just by being a part of a family with diabetes, they have often grown up with the same food likes and dislikes, not to mention the same lifestyles and commonalities as their parents and siblings? Yes, genetics can be a factor, but we are also what we learn. We are definitely products of those who raised us. If one really wishes to change, one needs to learn a different lifestyle and learn how to live in a healthier way. Change is by no means easy, for we are truly creatures of habit. However, when we are faced with such a deadly disease, we must never forget that we, as individuals, are worth more than that extra piece of cake or that sedentary lifestyle we live.

Many times people eat to compensate for a lack in life. Where quality of food is not met, people will eat more to compensate for what they are not receiving in their lives and diets. Often they will eat meals that are very high in *refined sugars* and *processed foods.* When one consumes these two types of foods, one will see two culprits to disease emerging. Not only is this a fundamental finding in diabetes, but it is a fundamental fact to most illnesses. This is truly why so many people are ill today.

HIGH BLOOD PRESURE:

Many factors contribute to high blood pressure, such as age, sex, family history, ethnicity, obesity, stress, and foods high in sodium and/or cholesterol. This disease's etiology is at times ninety percent unknown. Diet and lack of exercise play a large role when it comes to this condition. Quite often, I will see people with *Buddha bellies* or increased fat in their midsections and thighs, who also have high blood pressure. Here, what needs to be remembered, is that the human body was never created to carry such a weight. As human beings, we must be cognizant that when young we are conditioned by those who feed us. As we age, we become then products of our own choices. As a society today, people are content to sit in front of their televisions and computers, rather than go out for exercise and movement. With fast food on every corner and the mentality of, "I want what I want when I want it," it is no wonder this disease is growing at the rate it is.

To the skinny hypertensive, one will later read how inappropriate hydration can be a reason why one's blood pressure might be high.

SMOKING:

If you smoke, you will probably die of lung cancer or some other related disease like emphysema or chronic obstructive pulmonary disease (COPD). Although, this is a well-known fact, did you know that there are other underlying reasons for this problem? One does not need to be a rocket scientist to come to this conclusion. Nicotine is addictive. As with any other addiction, nicotine is a substitute for something that is missing in your life. Yet, people do give up and quit this deadly habit every day. This positive change is because "the addict" has finally come to love and believe in themselves. They have finally begun to address their financial, physical, emotional, and mental dependence, and have started to reclaim their lives. It does not matter whether one is addicted to alcohol, drugs, smoking, food, shopping, gambling, work, or sex. Overcoming an addiction is just a matter of true intimacy and honesty with one's self. It is important to understand the reasons for the mental dependency before the physical addiction can ever be addressed. Remember, it is most often the *underlying reasons* that cause us to injure ourselves.

DEPRESSION:

Many people have suffered at some time in their lives from this disease. It can be debilitating and can even cause paralysis in some people's lives if not corrected. The medical community states it is a disease brought on by either an imbalance of serotonin, norepinephrine, or both in the brain. Yet, even though these levels can be drawn, the diagnostic levels have falter when it comes to the accuracy of what the brain actually produces. That is why one will find psychiatrists often altering the dosages of these antidepressants and even changing the medications themselves. This is so they can attempt to get the upper hand on this condition. However, when doctors do this, they are certainly playing with the chemicals in your brain. We must remember, if we choose to play with Mother Nature, we will eventually pay a price.

For those people who feel these medications are helping them, so be it. However, if we do not look further into the causes of our problems, we will probably see this disease surface again.

I have seen many times how the power of the mind can take us to a place where we believe a certain pill can help us. It is this power of the mind over the body that often triggers dependency on these antidepressants. Could we ever be open enough with ourselves to realize that many circumstances of depression are much more than what we call a *chemical imbalance?* Many times, the problem lies within, in the emotions and mental burdens we carry. In depression, we see symptoms like sadness, grief, sorrow, fear, and anxiety. It is these emotions that will get our attention. It will be these emotions that will ultimately encourage us to seek out professional help.

When it comes to the issue of depression, I encourage counseling very much. This type of therapy can often offer the needed knowledge and support that is essential for a better outcome. Not only does this process allow one to become independent and accountable for the circumstances that have taken over their lives, but it also gives one the tools and principles to function on a higher level of well-being. When one functions with a sound mind, they will eventually and most often have a sound body.

Unfortunately, not all people are given the opportunity for counseling. Some adults do not want to seek it out due to the stigma attached to it. When issues such as abandonment and abuse are present, it is essential that one pursue this type of therapy not only to help understand their problems, but to have the appropriate guidance to uncover their true authentic self. Through this introspection, one can begin to address and overcome their issues of depression. If someone believes only in the quick fix of a pill to help them with this problem, then one most definitely has missed what is needed to get back their personal control of their life.

Only look to those who continue to struggle with depression while on these medications, or to those who have killed themselves while taking these pills. With good professional and personal support and insight, one can learn how to be emotionally sound. With positive attitudes, one can learn how to be proactive in the face of adversity. With *self-love, self-care, and self-esteem*, one can finally learn how to be comfortable within themselves, and truly understand the person they were meant to be.

HEART DISEASE:

Except in cases of structural damage or congenital abnormalities, many causes of heart disease have been overlooked or have taken less precedence when it comes to treating heart conditions.

While working in Los Angeles years ago, I remember taking a class on heart disease. One issue discussed was the topic of the *typical cardiac*. Here, the educator stated that most cardiac patients were usually *Type A personalities. They are the* must-do-it-right-type of people whose stress levels place a great demand on their hearts. Frequently, these cardiac patients were found to be working in the business world or in occupations that had very high levels of stress. Unhealthy eating habits, especially in the consumption of red meats and high cholesterol foods, were often seen. Addictions to alcohol and cigarettes were also reported. Today, people are more aware of these findings. However, what still remains as a concern is the consistency of stress or the rigors of one's lifestyle that affects the heart. For these people, it is most definitely a necessity for them to learn how to take a break and learn how to incorporate daily exercise, meditation and recreation into their lives. Learning to "stop and smell the roses" is exactly what one needs when it comes to preventing this heart-breaking disease.

We have all heard the expressions, "he died of a broken heart" or "what a great heart she has." When people talk this way, they are talking about emotions. When it comes to this vital organ, we should never forget this fact. Often with chronic sadness, grief, sorrow, and anger, we can see profound effects on the heart. Not only do these emotions affect the arteries, often they can damage the myocardium (the muscular tissue surrounding the heart) and the heart itself.

Another disease of the heart, which I believe needs discussion, is a condition known as atrial fibrillation. This is the most common cause of arrhythmias, or irregular heartbeat, and is frequently a factor seen in aging. Often if not treated, it can eventually decrease one's supply of blood and oxygen to all their vital organs. As a result, the heart does not pump correctly which ultimately can cause a problem of pooling and stagnation of the blood. When this occurs, there is the possibility of clot formation. Many conditions such as high blood pressure, overactive thyroid, valve disease, lung disease, stress, heart attacks and heart defects have been contributing factors of this condition.

Although it is true that a fibrillating heart can cause clots, the medical community approaches the treatment of this disease without any regard to the true underlying cause or emotional state of the individual patient. Instantly, the patient is placed on a possible life-long list of medications that will certainly affect their lives in many ways. Anti-arrhythmia drugs, blood thinners, aspirin, and possible anti-hypertensive combination medications are the treatment of choice. Naturally, the arrhythmia needs to be treated when it occurs, but what concerns me is how often doctors tend to neglect the other obvious causes leading to this disease. What needs to be addressed are stimulants like alcohol, coffee, nicotine, soda, diets high in red meat, and highly processed foods like sugar and refined flour, not to mention stress factors and medications taken by these patients. Have these causes been passed over or not even addressed at all before a treatment has been decided? The same is also true when we look at the proven overuse of pacemakers and other intra-cardiac devices. Yes, these devices regulate and keep the heart going, but could the use of these interventions have been avoided, if the medical community would have only listened to what the heart was truly trying to say?

Another question I have for physicians is how the use of these cardiac-specific drugs can, and most often will, affect the balance of electrolytes in our bodies? Two of these specific electrolytes are sodium and potassium. Both of these elements work together to maintain and regulate the total amount of water in the body helping to ensure proper body functions. If this delicate system becomes altered, as it can be with the use of many cardiac drugs, then we most certainly can have further problems related to these cardiac interventions.

So, if one is suffering from heart disease or any disease, one needs to make sure they have all the answers before they ever start playing with these types of medicines and devices. One needs to ask many questions and gather as much information as possible about other treatment options. This eventually will prevent many problems down the road with regard to one's health, finances, and most of all one's life.

LIVER DISEASE:

In order to understand exactly the extent of this disease, we must understand exactly what the liver does. This organ filters the blood while it excretes bile that helps digest fats. It helps the body save energy while it produces important proteins necessary to keep your blood from clotting. It metabolizes many medications while it stores various vitamins. It converts plasma proteins into amino acids, such as albumin. Please note: Albumin levels for many can be the single most important indicator of the health status of an individual. When levels of albumin are low, quite often one's risk of contracting a possible disease skyrockets. This occurs because the immune system is usually battling invasion of toxins and other infectious diseases. Anyone with continuous infections and illnesses should always have these levels tested.

When discussing the liver, we need also to recognize that this organ also regulates and breaks down nutrients between the blood and the body's cells. When this organ does not function, we will often see the common problem known as malnutrition. Many think this is just not eating enough, but it is more complex than that. It is often the lack of eating *quality* food, combined with the inappropriate *quantity* of certain foods and harmful drinks that we consume that will allow this disease to develop.

Remember, when we eat processed food (dead food), we permit the liver to become lifeless and clogged with toxins. We see not only sickness, but we see the failure of this organ to function correctly. Alcoholism, drug abuse, and overuse of medications, and eating poorly are only a few causes of this disease. If one chooses to abuse drugs and eat improperly, then they must remember; that they are the responsible culprits for the decay of this organ, as well as many other organs in their bodies.

RENAL DISEASE:

This disease is often seen with diabetes and high blood pressure. Like the liver, this organ filters toxins and waste products from the blood and eventually from our bodies. When the kidneys do not function, we will quite often again see abnormal electrolyte imbalances. Thus, we will find our bodies retaining fluids or even having heart arrhythmias or other muscular problems. This is usually related to lower levels of calcium and sodium with higher levels of phosphorous in the blood. With increased phosphate levels we will see symptoms like itching, bone changes and muscular cramps. With renal disease, we will also see potassium levels that can be elevated, but they will vary according to the body's ability to conserve this element. Often edema of the ankle's, lungs and heart (congestive heart failure) can be seen with this disease. Added to these problems, we can often observe elevated urea (products of protein decomposition) levels, which will eventually exhibit itself in symptoms of vomiting, dehydration, weight loss, nocturnal urination and blood in the urine. Also what is seen are increased creatine levels that signal kidney damage usually related to prolonged levels of hyperglycemia often seen in severe diabetes.

When the kidney's flow is disrupted, we can also see signs and symptoms of renal disease. When people have surgery, we need to realize that anesthesia will slow down the flow of the body. When one overdoses or takes foreign chemicals like antibiotics (especially strong and heavy-duty ones) or chemotherapy agents, we can also see many adverse effects to this organ. We must recognize that when we choose to overuse medications, we will present our bodies with many more possible problems in the future.

Many times, we need to ask ourselves if taking these medications is worth what it is eventually "costing us." In addition to drugs and their immediate effects, we need to remember the following facts. When it comes to the liver, kidney and the rest of our bodies, we need to understand that the food we choose to eat, the beverages we choose to drink, and the pills we choose to take will often be the reasons for why we are sick. Let us never forget that most diseases certainly will occur, if we continue to remain oblivious to the effects of what we choose to consume.

CHAPTER 4

LET'S LOOK AT GOVERNMENT

Government is here to serve the citizens, not for the citizens to serve the government. Today, government is not for the people or by the people. It is above the people. It is a big business with too many self-serving individuals within who do not do what they said they would. No matter what their party affiliations are, many of these politicians are not upholding the fundamental tenets of this country. They have chosen not to be accountable for their abusive and wasteful ways. They continue to put their need for power and money above the needs of its people. Here, we must ask, *"Are we, the American people, responsible for what this government has chosen to do to itself and to this country?"*

Today, many people are finally realizing that they are no longer functioning with the possibility of hope, but rather they are only functioning on a level of survival. If we look to the poor, we will see that they have been enabled by this government to stay at the level where the middle class is now heading. Only look to the enormous unemployment rates and to the benefits that they offer. Are people moving forward or are they just remaining stagnant in the life they are *allowed* to live?

The expression that the rich are getting richer and the poor are getting poorer is entirely appropriate in these times. With this said, we need to remain aware that many people in our country are too dependent on government subsidies in order to live. These benefits are not only grossly over-utilized, but they have stifled people's abilities to grow in a healthy and prosperous way. As we become dependent, we lose our fundamental rights and liberties. This fact should never be taken lightly. If we do not become aware of the extreme consequences of this situation, we will wake up one day and realize that our freedoms are gone and that government is progressively moving to own us.

They have threatened to cut our Medicare and Social Security benefits. As American citizens, most of us have worked hard in our lives for this coverage, and we have paid for these benefits. Does government not realize that these benefits belong to us, and it is our money they have chosen to mismanage and throw away? Here, we must also remember that this is the time when the baby boomers, some twenty-six percent of the population, are reaching retirement and are in need of these benefits. How ironic that these cutbacks occur now, when the money is so desperately needed by so many.

Is it not this government that has allowed so many people to remain in this country after they have broken our laws? Did you know that Congress could eradicate the problem of illegal immigration very easily with just one proposal? In addition, ratification by state conventions would also eliminate this problem by law. Do we really need to reiterate that it is against the law to be here illegally? It is as plain and simple as that. Do we really need to protest such a fact? A law is a law and we need to make sure that our laws are enforced. America, it is *you* who needs to respond to this, and now is the time to get control of these matters.

If you search the Internet for the percentage of illegal people covered under welfare, Medicare, Medi-Cal, food stamps, low income housing, and unemployment benefits, you will discover that there are very few accurate statistics. This is because of poor quality control, inadequate reviews, and misrepresentation by illegal aliens and government combined. Overall, illegal immigration has allegedly cost the American taxpayer $110-$300 billion annually. What contributes to these enormous costs? Approximately, forty-three percent of food stamps, fifty-eight percent of welfare, and forty-one percent of unemployment benefits go to illegal aliens and their families. These percentages were from 2006, and are most likely much higher due to such factors as crimes of violence, schooling, deportation, and other issues not mentioned.

How ironic is it that this government cannot handle its own accounting of this issue? Although these benefits have been set up to help the American citizen, those who have entered our country illegally are the people who are benefiting greatly from them.

Since government benefits are derived from our tax dollars, illegal immigrants who are receiving benefits cause higher taxes to cover these programs. With this fact known, one becomes more fully aware of where some of our tax dollars are going, and why certain healthcare costs are skyrocketing the way they are. If we were ever to be able to restrict these government benefits so that only legal citizens would receive them, then and only then, would these programs be there in greater amounts for its American citizens. This country is in desperate need of these benefits, and, again, this government needs to be there for its *citizens.*

Many illegal immigrants are paid under the table. Some say this figure is over fifty percent. Since these workers do not always contribute to payroll taxes, this places just another burden on this country. Much of an illegal emigrant's money is sent out of the country to their extended families. Here, I am not questioning the right of people to do what they want with their money, but I am questioning how much money is actually leaving this country?

Another fact we must also look at with reference to government services and illegal immigrants is *"anchor"* or *"jackpot"* babies. These are babies born in the United States to illegal immigrants. Some 380,000 children were born to illegal immigrant parents in 2005. Here, the American taxpayer paid for over ninety-seven percent of all costs of these births. As of 2010, statistics show over 400,000 new arrivals for that year. Just by crossing the border, illegal parents have given to their children *our* inalienable rights, not to mention eighteen more years of ongoing benefits. It only takes having a U.S. address and a utility bill to qualify an illegal mother to get birth-related care in California's version of Medicaid, not to mention those who do not pay. It appears breaking the law has given illegal immigrants many rights for the many wrongs that have been done. We need also to realize that multiple children will create financial gains for illegal households. Not only does this produce future financial problems for the states and country, it creates legal ramifications for legalized children of illegal parents. At what cost is our country paying for illegal immigration?

An option that government has talked about is placing financial penalties against the illegal immigrants, or on the employers who have hired them. However, does this not just put money back into the government's pocket? Paying these penalties is just a very cheap and easy way to buy one's way out of a wrongdoing. If one is illegal, they should not receive any benefits.

Now, do not get me wrong. I believe there are many wonderful people who are responsible, law-abiding immigrants who are illegal, but they must be encouraged to pursue citizenship in an honest and lawful way. They most certainly deserve to obtain all they dream about, but they need to realize if deferential treatment is given out of default, it will only create animosity and chaos. This country cannot continue to burden itself with the problems of other countries, when we ourselves are drowning.

In these difficult times, we must learn to take care of ourselves before we can ever take care of others. When the plane is going down, we need to take care of ourselves first. This is called survival. If this is not taken seriously, we will never return to a place where we can help others as we once could.

We are told that our economy would collapse if people were forced to return to their native lands. This is not totally accurate. Billions of dollars would be saved, not to mention the amount of jobs that would be available for American citizens. Illegal immigrants are servicing approximately eight and a half million jobs as we speak. Close to eleven million Americans are looking for work. Compare these numbers. They say people would not work for such low wages, but let us realize that less than two percent of the illegal population is actually picking crops. Many illegal aliens are working in jobs that many citizens would and could work in. Only when we realize this, will we ever see more jobs returning to our citizens. It will only be when we see American citizens returning to work, that we will ever see a level of self-preservation begin to occur once again in this country. The dependency of the people on government subsidies would decrease greatly, which would allow us to, once again, find our way back to employment, freedom, and hope. If one remains dependent on the system, they will not only lose their own power and control, but they will ultimately lose their own sense of self. This is especially necessary for one's own growth and strength. We should never forget this very important and fundamental principle of life.

Another concern about government is its own statement about immigration reform. They stated, "This country really can't expect us to deport over 11 million people who are here illegally?" The answer to this is... yes, we can. It is government's job to protect its people and obey the laws of this country. If government has been so negligent for such a long time and has not done their job correctly, then it truly is their responsibility to fix this problem. It should not be done in the easiest way, but rather in the most honest and accurate way. Is this not what we pay government to do? Most American citizens are not happy with how government is handling this issue, and government needs to listen to its people?

Another issue that needs discussion concerns people who have come to this country *legally*. Sometimes without ever working, legal immigrants receive benefits like welfare, housing, and food stamps. There once was a time when immigrants coming to America or bringing family members to America, were responsible for supporting themselves and their families. This included housing, food, healthcare, and transportation. This is not true anymore. With reference to this issue, what government needs to learn is to have more precise statistics of legal immigrants and new citizens who are on benefits like unemployment, welfare, and workmen's compensation. Stricter regulations and evaluations need to be instituted and those who know that they truly do not belong on these subsidies need to stop their abusive ways. Here, what is often found is that many people would rather utilize these resources than ever look for work.

As a nation, we are well aware that it is easier to take advantage and lie to these government and state agencies than to really address the actual issue, which is honesty to oneself. This only adds to the many reasons why we see this country heading towards bankruptcy. To those who utilize the systems and abuse the laws, it is necessary for each person to look at their actions and take responsibility. What many have done is not right or deserving. It is a pure deception not only to oneself, but also to this country.

As for the government, it is essential that they examine their issues and realize the wrongs they have done with reference to their greed and lack of accountability. Government must understand how their actions have hindered the growth of America. This is not only true for the future of our children, but for the future of our healthcare. The government needs to act with integrity toward the citizens it serves and once again rule by its laws. In this time, we need leaders that will look at the real issues and who will believe in what this country is capable of achieving. Government, you are not listening again to your people. You have answered only to the *power* for which you wish to attain. When there is no longer money, we can no longer spend, nor can we pay higher taxes for those who do not have. If we were to give an allowance to a child and they did not learn to use it wisely, we would be fools to give them more

If this government were an individual, by now they would be broke. Guess what? They are. Is government so oblivious and above it all that they do not see this crater that is oozing with fire? Government now has the chance to redeem itself, but only if they rise to this challenge and learn from their mistakes. If they do not, they will never regain the respect and support of the people who trusted them to govern. It is imperative that government statistics be complete and that financial accounting be open and in order for this country to see the facts. Although, officials claim that we are seventeen trillion dollars in debt, if our government continues to do what they are doing, they will remain playing its citizens for fools. Only when government learns to speak the truth, will we ever have the correct commitment that a strong country needs.

With government now more involved in healthcare, we must address this issue of their interference. The bottom line is government does not belong in healthcare. Healthcare belongs in the hands of the people who work within the profession itself. Is it not preposterous, how government has found its way into a field of which it has so little knowledge? How can government ever think it can handle healthcare when it cannot even handle itself? We need only to look at the disarray of Congress and the president to see the lack of cohesiveness, leadership and productivity as they govern. Does this not speak for the reality of this situation?

With the enactment of the new healthcare bill, it is worrisome that government has placed itself in a situation with a piece of legislation that many of its constituents and legislators have neither read, nor understand. The goal is to provide care to all, but is this really the most important issue? Is not quality of care more important than quantity? Before this problem can be approached, the following facts need to be discussed.

We must remember when it comes to healthcare; it is *big business* and with big business, comes *big bucks*. America, do not kid yourself; the government is in this for the money. With money comes power and with power comes control. Concisely, this is why government wishes to have its hands in your healthcare.

With this being understood, let us look at two federal statutes to show exactly how inefficiently this government runs healthcare. We shall look at the Emergency Medical Treatment and Labor Act (EMTALA) and the Health Insurance Portability and Accountability Act (HIPAA). Although both these were enacted by federal agencies to provide guidelines to protect the patients, many times they show their own hypocrisy and shortcomings when it comes to the protection they provide.

To substantiate these findings, let us discuss EMTALA. One of EMTALA's regulations states that any hospital with an emergency room must give any person a medical screening and stabilize them regardless of a person's ability to pay. This statement in and of itself has led hospitals to enormous and outstanding financial burdens. We know, if anyone were ever to be unstable, we would never put these people back out into the streets, but when people come to the emergency room for convenience, we have a very serious and expensive problem that we are confronting.

I believe it is unconscionable that without proper

identification, many people come and go without any means to pay for the many services rendered. Both government and hospitals are aware of this issue. When I see patients coming to emergency rooms by way of ambulance for a common cold or fever and they say that they did not have a car to get them there, or that their spouse was not at home, then we most assuredly see this dilemma. When patients say they could not use the clinic, I need to question this statement, because at the clinic one might have to pay something for treatment, while in the ER people can often come and go without any payment.

Many times, people come to an ER and give one name, and if it is, later determined surgery is necessary, that name suddenly changes. Again, we have another problem. I ask, "What is really going on here, and how much more abuse of this system can we tolerate?" I do not ever remember going into a store, choosing an item I needed, then proceeding to the checkout counter and saying, "Sorry, I don't have the money, but I'll take it anyway." Since when do we think, *I will get it for free* refers to healthcare?

If government wishes to make all these laws, then I say they also need to change things with regard to illegal and fraudulent practices by those who utilize the system. It would be easy to solve this problem. Just have all people present citizenship papers with authentic identification (maybe by way of E-Verify or by a person's paystub). When it comes to this specific issue of authenticity, this would also take care of the many prejudicial concerns that so many people are worried about.

When talking about laws and regulations with regard to hospitals, here is another question. Would it not be good to eliminate most of government agencies that have cost billions to the taxpayers and have cost healthcare financially and emotionally? Most assuredly, many credible people in healthcare are capable of doing this job just as well if not better. Ultimately, this would eliminate government from continuing to pay extravagant costs for its many bureaucratic ways.

Often, we find government placing steep financial penalties onto hospitals when they are not compliant. Would it not be better to reward hospitals that show good compliance and governing, rather than just to penalize them? This would help hospitals with increased financial burdens to maintain themselves, while it would also promote competition within the industry itself. If we wish to cut costs in healthcare, this is a perfect place to begin. This is called *self-regulation*. Actually, this is what is essential for any successful outcome in a business. Healthcare is an industry that is highly capable of managing itself and wishes very much to do so.

Now, let us look at HIPAA. These are laws and regulations once again written by government. They are the rules that are followed by doctors, hospitals, and other healthcare providers. They help ensure that all medical records, billing, and patient accounts meet certain consistent standards with regard to handling and privacy. In two words, it is *privacy* and *protection* for the patient, but some of these rules are utterly ridiculous and inconsistent.

Recently, in California, HIPAA proceeded to fine a hospital for multiple violations at a cost of $50,000 per violation. These penalties were for violations of privacy of individual patients' information and for overcrowding. They stated, "Patients being treated in hallways had no privacy, and that all people belonged in their own cubicles in the emergency room." Let me ask anyone who has ever been in an emergency room or hospital room: have you not accidentally overheard about another patient's issues while you were a patient? Since when does a privacy curtain really grant someone privacy? Privacy is still being violated and this travesty of legislation and assumptions by government policies is not really answering these issues. To complicate matters, we find that most waiting rooms are filled to over-sized capacity, and unable to accommodate the needs of its people. Once again, the hospital is at fault for not providing to its patients proper access to care and treatment in a reasonable time, and another $50,000 goes to government.

Truthfully, in healthcare, do we really have the ability to know how many people will be knocking on our hospital doors? Which is more important: penalties, or trying to care for the patients the best we can? Although intentions may be to protect and provide for the patient's welfare, it comes down to those who really understand and work every day in this war zone called "healthcare". If hospitals were able to control themselves with fewer interventions by government, not only would cost go down, but also hospitals could finally be able to address internal issues without interference. If a hospital produced quality care rather than just provide for quantity, it would then be able to speak for itself. When hospitals perform in quality ways, we will see patients returning. What this is called is *competition,* and this word is something very important in any business.

When ObamaCare initially came out, it amazed me how the hospitals became inundated with people coming to the emergency room stating, "I am here for the free health care." If we think giving healthcare to over 30 to 50 million more people will be cheaper, how will this actually occur, if not at the cost to the American taxpayer? Not only will quality decrease, but also we will see many professionals leaving this type of care. We must acknowledge this fact, if we ever wish to move in a more productive and realistic way toward producing more efficient healthcare. This country is in desperate need of reform, but what is being presented to the American public is *not* the correct answer.

Another instance of government intervention in healthcare was the development of DRGs in the early 1980's. These coding systems were designed to provide practice information to administrators of hospitals, and were utilized to alter the behaviors and spending by its doctors, surgeons, and medical staff. This program limited the share of hospital revenues derived from Medicare and eventually Medi-Cal. A certain diagnosis determines how a provider is actually paid by utilizing these codes. Although its founders were not government officials, the coding system was ultimately supported by the Centers for Medicare and Medi-Cal (CMS), which are both government-based programs.

Although the pilot study of this system's effects was *doubtful* and *failed* initially in the state of New Jersey, the government chose to implement it anyway. Here, for the first time, the federal government gained the upper hand in its financial relationship with the medical community. This enactment created a shift in the balance of political and economic power between the provider of medical care (hospitals and physicians) and by those who paid for it. (Here, it is important to note that some people believe that it is the government and the insurance companies who pay for healthcare, but in actuality it is the taxpayers who really pays).When this venture occurred, this is the way government and the insurance companies entered into the healthcare industry *together*. This was one of the most significant changes in healthcare policies since the passage of Medicare and Medi-Cal in 1965, that went virtually unnoticed by the general public. Initially, it was somewhat cost effective, but it is not any longer. It is partially due to this enactment that we now see healthcare providers dictated to with regard to what is allowed in the care of their patients and clients. Today, it is these restrictions of services that are permitted by laws that have altered the care that is offered to people. This is the *basic reason* why healthcare has changed so drastically and has declined in this country. Once again, government stepped in and enforced their beliefs on the way healthcare should be delivered. How ironic that these prices have soared even with this enactment. How interesting that we find many patients stating that healthcare is not the way it once was, nor will it ever be again.

Being personally involved with government agencies and insurance companies, I wish to share some personal situations of my own experience as a nurse that shows how inefficiency and fiscally wasteful government and insurance companies can be.

While working at a government facility in California in 1985, the head of accounting shared with me that in just this one facility, approximately seventy-seven million dollars had been allegedly lost in just one fiscal year. The money could not be accounted for, nor was this situation ever investigated. This information was from a very dedicated and concerned employee of this facility, who worked there for over twenty-five years. Another personal experience that speaks for itself was a job that I worked at in the state of Maine. This was an insurance company where I did chart reviews. Many of these specific reviews were for Medicare reimbursements. In this company, a pilot study was done, which ended up costing more than $660,000. Halfway through this study, this private insurance company realized the conclusion was not going the way they wanted, so they just abruptly ended it. No data released, no data kept. I ask, "Who is paying for this awful waste?" At this same company, there was even more waste with reference to the expedition of the paperwork.

As we know, documentation is of the utmost importance when it comes to healthcare. However, in this facility, employees were encouraged not to read all of the elaborate documentation, to facilitate the speed of processing for reimbursement. Diagnosis and ultimate care given were the only things required for the approval of these payments. Hence, if this elaborate documentation was often overlooked, why does it need to be done in the first place? An easy checklist would give healthcare the same results. If one is truly concerned with why medical costs are so high and why we are going bankrupt in this system, I believe government and the insurance industry needs to answer some questions. They need to tell all of America, where our money has really gone. They need to explain fully all the wastes for all of these years. I believe this is called an audit, which the government does quite often with reference to its own citizens. If the government can show us where every dollar has gone, we will finally have the answers this country truly deserves.

As American citizens, we must also realize that it is not only this lack of accountability by government and other agencies that have let us down, but it is our own personal accountability as well. We must realize that our lack of following these ongoing concerns of this country has also allowed these poor choices to be made.

People today are so overwhelmed with their own personal and financial problems that they sometimes continue to remain oblivious to the activities and affairs of government and other involved agencies. While more people are now recognizing these issues, numerous problems remain that we as Americans need to address. Although personal problems like unemployment and financial matters are still present in our lives, it is of utmost importance that we begin to educate ourselves. This education includes becoming aware of the pertinent issues of this country and finding the truth. However, do not look to the media. Many times, big corporations, which have too many vested interests, own them. Furthermore, it is important that we become involved. This is not only for our own sake, but also for the sake of our children as well as our country. If we choose to remain unaware of what is actually occurring, than we can only say that we are also culprits of these issues. We must ultimately ask ourselves if we are partially responsible for this downfall of America.

A classic example of this is what has occurred with the new healthcare reform bill. At first, many citizens dreamed how wonderful this free healthcare would be. Now many know it is not so. When we look at these proposed new benefits, we can see that nothing is for free. What we will see is not only taxes rising to pay for this bill, but we will see many of our benefits becoming profoundly limited. The icing on this cake may look good, but wait until one takes a bite of this cake. To this finding, let us now inspect some of these issues of this new reform.

First, Congress and staff committee members are exempt from this mandated healthcare while the average citizen has fewer options. Although, this issue is still disputable, we need to consider the actions of this potential enactment and realize that Congress has most certainly attempted to place itself on a different level to the average citizen. Second, remember once again that placing approximately 30 to 50 million more people on this bill will never make healthcare cheaper. Third, this bill will eventually cause increased unemployment because the employer will not be able to pay these increased premiums and penalties for their employees. Lastly, government has mortgaged us to the tune of millions, if not billions of dollars in order to enact this bill. Then, they have the *audacity* to lecture us on accountability for this myth rather than the reality it presents. How easy it is for them to throw our money away, not to mention the healthcare we need.

Another example of government's pretense of good intentions is when we look at the issue of immigration reform. It is not actual compassion that is at the heart of this proposed reform, but rather it is the needed revenue and possible future votes from illegal citizens. We need to remember that some of these illegal immigrants do pay state and federal taxes, not to mention over $9 billion a year to Social Security. In 2007, the President's Council of Economic Advisors cited that the average immigrant pays a net of $80,000 more in taxes than what they will ever collect in government services. Therefore, it is important to be mindful that this perceived compassion is not really representative of what America speaks for, but rather for the greed of some government officials for the taxes, votes, and power that they wish to obtain.

When I look at us as a country involved with other countries, fighting for what they call world peace, I see the need to step back and realize that peace must be established at home first. Before we can ever go elsewhere, we must first take care of ourselves. Just look at our country: people still fighting for decent healthcare, still fighting against racial discrimination, people still living on the streets, losing their jobs and their homes, people not receiving what they need and what they have earned, and most important, people still trying to be heard. Yes, we need to look deeply and realize we are a country that can no longer give as we used to.

As a country, it is time to take off our blindfolds. We cannot be ignorant any longer. We need to take back our country, and this needs to occur now. Once again, we need to be a country with honesty, integrity and decency for all. This government needs to be examined for its abuse of, and its lack of, compliance with constitutional law. This action needs to be demanded by its people in an organized and peaceful way. Congress cannot do it, because many members of the legislative body are also culprits. Their own questionable and suspicious actions have shown that we can no longer trust any of them despite the good efforts of some. Look at how many legislators are now speaking out and exposing the existing government corruption. Did they not know of these issues before?

We need to realize that action by citizens needs to be initiated state by state, with each state's people heavily involved. Here, compliance by the American people is most assuredly the main ingredient for change. The only remedy for this is for the people to finally take action. We must return America to a standard of living that will be one of growth and health for its people. Only when this is accomplished, can we reclaim the pride we once had. It needs to be a movement based on virtues and morals, not corruption and deception. It should be one of reform, not revolt. No, I am not a radical, but I am a concerned citizen who is tired of all the worthless rhetoric.

In the following chapters, we will look at two industries that play a large part in healthcare. We will learn not only how these industries really work, but who actually pays the eventual costs that these multi-billion-dollar conglomerates make. While these industries are here to provide for and protect us, we must always remain aware they have also taken much from their captive consumers.

CHAPTER 5

LET'S LOOK AT PHARMACEUTICAL COMPANIES

A row of bottles on my shelf
Caused me to analyze myself.
One yellow pill I have to pop
Goes to my heart so it won't stop.
A little white one that I take
Goes to my hands so they won't shake.
The blue ones that I use a lot
Tell me I am happy when I'm not.
The purple pill goes to my brain
And tells me that I have no pain.
The capsules tell me not to wheeze,
Or cough or choke or even sneeze.
The red ones, smallest of them all
Go to my blood so I won't fall
The orange ones, very big and bright
Prevent my leg cramps in the night.

Such an array of brilliant pills
Helping to cure all kinds of ills.
But what I'd really like to know
Is what tells each one where to go!

--Anonymous

Although this author is unknown, I am most grateful for these words of wisdom. Not only are drugs utilized abundantly, but they have also placed a tremendous financial burden on the people of this country and of the world. Drugs may be an easy way to fix a problem, but they are not always a permanent solution to the many illnesses of today. Whether they cause side effects or synergistic effects (how each drug interacts with one another), drugs often present reactions that damage our bodies. Granted, drugs have their place when utilized correctly on a short-term basis, but when a pill is a necessity for long-term use, we need to look closely at its use and the potential for abuse.

As of 2009, pharmaceutical manufacturers are the third most profitable industry in the country. The pharmaceutical industry makes over $600 billion a year. Pfizer's executive and CEO made $1.7 million in 2011, and received compensation worth a total of

$18.12 million. For some other CEO's, they have received up to and over $30 million in profits for just one year's earnings. Thus, we need only to count the many salaries, bonuses and stock options of these mega billion dollar companies, and we have found a place where much of the profits have gone in this business.

This industry claims that most of its money goes into research and development. However, this is not as accurate as one may think. It has been estimated that two and one half times as much money goes into marketing and administration than is spent on research. So, how does this development and research of a drug actually work?

Drugs have a patent for approximately ten years. At the end of the ninth year, many times the pharmaceutical companies will take out the chemicals that work in the first drug and place them into a second, newer drug. This version then has a new patent. Although some research has been done to extract the old and reform it into a new product, very little change to the drug has actually taken place. Thus, a new drug, a more expensive drug has been created that is really just an updated version of the old one.

If we look at the research of antibiotics today, we will find with the exception of two pharmaceutical companies, that this kind of research is virtually dead. The reason for this is that antibiotics are not as profitable as medication for cancer, heart, and high blood pressure. This reality leaves people who are being treated for superbugs and drug resistant diseases in a very helpless and precarious place. It actually is leaving this country open to a health crisis that could be of epic proportions down the road. Today, bacterial and parasitic diseases are the second leading cause of death worldwide. Why is this problem of death and dying occurring? Once again, because of the greed and lack of accountability of these drug companies at the expense of the patients.

Over the years, pharmaceutical companies have created many drugs that have been known to have many adverse reactions or side effects. Let us look at some of these questionable drugs to see what they actually do and how they have fared with regards to their many adverse effects.

The first drug is Avandia. This is a medication for Type II Diabetes. It works by increasing the body's sensitivity to insulin, while it helps to lower the blood sugar and keeps it under control. People who take Avandia are often seen at higher risk for heart attacks, kidney problems and other serious complications. While Avandia has been linked to possibly 80,000 patient deaths and caused heart attacks and strokes in some 200,000 people, it still remains on the market and is readily available to the public. The FDA examined some of these claims for this drug, and responded by adding a warning label that stated that the pharmaceutical trial was inadequately designed and was not fully conducted to prove the drug was completely safe. Recently, Avandia has been removed from use in Europe. In October 2011, the FDA was to remove this drug in America, but as of August, 2012, it remains on the shelves, alongside Actos (another diabetic drug) that has been linked to bladder cancer and tumors. Here, we must ask, why consumers are not being protected immediately.

Another drug of importance that needs to be mentioned is Coumadin. This drug is a blood thinner. Prescribed to prevent clot formation, it is often used by patients with atrial fibrillation. I must warn everyone to be careful with this drug. Since many patients are on Coumadin, I find that more education really needs to be done when speaking about this drug. I find that when I meet a person taking Coumadin, I rarely have to ask them if they are on this medication. Why, because one only needs to look at the black and blue bruises often seen on their fragile skin to realize that this drug has already shown it's self. Although many people say they do not feel well when they are utilizing this medication, patients continue to take it anyway. The two reasons they give for this are: their doctors told them that they have to take it, and if they do not, they will probably develop clots and die.

However, if patients find themselves bleeding from their stomachs, rectums, noses, eyes, or if one's skin looks terrible, they had better start listening to what their body is saying. While the reason for taking Coumadin is to prevent complications, the side effects from this drug have already shown its own complications. There are alternative treatments with no side effects, like taking willow bark, eating greens, and taking enzymes to replace the use of this questionable drug. People should really try to look into these different options with the guidance of their practitioners.

Another class of drugs that needs to be looked into is medications known as "statins". These drugs are prescribed to treat high cholesterol. Statins have been promoted to prevent heart attack and stroke. Today, many doctors believe these drugs are one of the greatest breakthroughs in medicine, but I disagree. As a nurse, I have seen too many people with side effects from these medications. Statins have killed and injured more people than what the government or pharmaceutical companies have admitted. This was quoted in a January 2012, edition of USA Today, "The side effects such as liver and kidney damage, memory loss and muscle weakness and links to diabetes are only some of these drugs' destructive side effects." Although studies are still being done on this drug, we need to ask why this drug continues to remain on the market, when not all the questions about its uses have been answered. If you do not feel well on this medication, remember that your body is talking to you.

Other noteworthy drugs used often today are incredible amounts of pain medications, sleep aids, and antidepressants. Society is developing an extreme dependency on these medicines. These medications can have a profound effect on one's well being. If these drugs are inappropriately prescribed and utilized freely, our society will be creating yet another profound addiction problem for itself.

When talking about drugs, we must never forget the Federal Drug Administration (FDA). As many people know, the FDA is supposed to protect us, the consumer. It was originally designed to monitor different products and devices for safety reasons. It was intended to control against any unwanted side effects from the industry's products. If this is so, then why do so many private and class action lawsuits occur? Why, then, are so many people being compensated for the serious legal and lethal implications of these drugs?

The FDA and the pharmaceutical companies have on their boards and panels many lawyers, doctors, and politicians who have a vested interest in the backing of these pharmaceutical companies. It is not only a job with a paycheck, but it is a job with incentives and rewards conducive to their work. Although at times these agencies do make good recommendations, we must be aware of the many oversights that do occur. So, the next time you go to pay for a prescription, realize the money you spend is most definitely going somewhere, but that somewhere is not necessarily funding research and development. Only ask why this country pays so much more than any other country for prescription drugs. Don't be surprised, if you find that it is because of regulations set up by the FDA, pharmaceutical companies, lobbyist, and the insurance companies themselves. So when you questions these findings just remember: Why should these agencies care about improving their products or reducing their prices when they have us supporting this multi-billion dollar business?

Before leaving this discussion of these pharmaceutical companies, I want to mention the television advertisements for these drugs. As the commercial ends, we are given a long list of side effects. Is this to protect us, the consumer, or is it to protect this industry? Just another question you might want to ask this lucrative big business, if you ever get the chance.

DIARIES OF A MAD NURSE

CHAPTER 6

LET'S LOOK AT THE HEALTH INSURANCE INDUSTRY AND HEALTHCARE ITSELF

The health insurance industry insists rising costs are to blame for runaway premiums. However, they also state, that rate hikes are surpassing the growth of medical costs, wages and overall inflation. Which statement is correct? Only by exploring this insurance industry itself and by looking at healthcare and its relationship to this industry, will we find the truth. The following will answer these questions.

In 2010, the four largest for-profit health insurance companies recorded huge profit gains in the *first quarter* of the year; Aetna, Cigna, United Healthcare, and WellPoint reported a combined net income of $3.2 billion. This was a thirty-one percent leap from the previous year. At a gathering of stockholders and executives of the insurance market, the CEO of one of these big companies stated, "People needing health care can't afford anything other than our low-based health plans. Because of this people will have to pay out of pocket to see a doctor or just to fill a prescription. Since this kind of plan is profitable, it is spreading like wildfire." He also went on to say, "People in the insurance industry are doing quite well." To this, I can only say, "Good job, big guy."

Between 2000 and 2008, healthcare premiums have increased ninety-seven percent. In 2009, economists stated that healthcare costs are close to $2.4 trillion, and can reach $4 trillion by the year 2016. As consumers, we pay for healthcare either through insurance or directly with our own money. This is known as *private sector spending*. When we speak of public funding on the other hand, we must understand that this kind of funding comes from tax dollars that federal, state and local governments use to pay for programs like Medicare and Medicaid. Today, these programs account for almost one out of every five dollars that government spends. It will be closer to every one out of three dollars by 2040.

As of 2009, insurance companies were paid twenty-eight percent by government (fourteen percent Medicaid and fourteen percent Medicare).

The private sector paid sixty-one percent while the remaining percent was paid out of pocket. (Fifty-seven percent of this was through employment based revenues). Studies show that from January 2009, to March 2010, fifty-eight percent of private-sector-based enrollments were falling by as much as 2.8 million Americans. This is a staggering figure. Since, employers pay approximately seventy-five percent of most employee health insurance premiums, we can see why these increased premiums have forced so many employers to stop sponsoring healthcare plans for their employees and their families.

The average cost of an insurance premium is $13,000 per family when paid by an employer. As employees, we pay approximately one quarter of this amount. Also, note that seven out of ten Americans who have some form of health insurance get it through an employer. In 2007, statistics showed that eight in ten uninsured people came from working families. Therefore, while eighty-six million people continue to have insurance, it is because they are paying higher premiums and out-of-pocket costs. Combined with member reductions and cuts in these employer sponsored plans, these *buy downs* as they are known in the industry are making many shareholders and executives in insurance companies very happy and quite rich.

These statistics will reinforce just how much healthcare actually costs the American public. As of 2009, sixty percent of bankruptcy filings in the United States have been because of medical expenses. The U.S. pays two and a half times as much on healthcare per capita than any other country. Yet, we rank in the thirty-eighth percentile in life expectancy, which equals 78.2 years of age. Surprisingly, other statistics show that adults only get fifty-five percent of the recommended care for the enormous amount of money being spent. Seventy-five percent of our costs are from patients with chronic diseases like heart, lung, diabetes, and cancer, while fifty percent of all healthcare spending pays for the care received by only five percent of the population.

Statistical studies also show an estimated 98,000 Americans die every year as a result of medical errors that have been linked to the healthcare that is available. Over 547, 000 people die yearly from cancer. Over 600,000 people die every year from heart disease as of 2011. Diabetes, the seventh leading cause of death in the U.S., kills approximately 180,000 people yearly. In 2011, over 443,000 people died from smoking. Thus, despite all the money we spend, often people do not get what they need. Only ask the people living below poverty level if they have more problems with the quality of their care than do the people with higher incomes.

Other factors that affect premiums are loss of a job or a change in employment. Also, note that family coverage stops because of factors such as advanced age or leaving school. Although ObamaCare has addressed some of these issues in its new reform, we must never forget that government does not belong in this industry. It does not belong in a business that already has too many regulations placed on it.

Today, twenty-six states have *no* regulatory authority to modify unreasonable rate hikes in the individual and small group markets. Most insurance companies have built near monopoly powers when it comes to this. Both healthcare and the insurance companies still have not restrained enough of their costs to prove that they can remedy this issue. Although trying, they are still wasteful and inefficient when it comes to complex billing and paperwork and its high administrative costs.

Are we getting our money's worth? Of course not! We have all seen how more money does not always get us more value. Consider uninsured Americans. Uninsured people are nearly eight times more likely to skip healthcare because they can't afford it. That means, we do not see them until their conditions worsen and they need to be treated in emergency rooms and hospitals. These services cost more than visits to a doctor's office. About half of uninsured adults with chronic health conditions go without recommended healthcare or medicine because of the cost. Thus, the only way the insurance companies drive down medical costs has been to stop insuring unhealthy people and this is exactly what has occurred in the industry. Thank God, this issue is finally being addressed, but that is far from why we should agree with ObamaCare. These pre-existing conditions prevent many from obtaining insurance, as well as other questionable issues of this industry. This is not to say that insurance companies are evil, it just means that they need some way to make these large profits. Otherwise, how else could they ever cover the costs of sales, marketing, underwriting, and other administrative expenses?

One last issue to be discussed when it comes to insurance companies is that of competition. In this one word, *competition*, we find a working solution to the issue of insurance premiums and of the other problems within this industry. As mentioned before, insurance regulations are mandated by state legislation. When states finally relinquish this hold on insurance companies, only then will we see premiums decrease. At present, there is very little competition in this industry, and therefore no motivation to keep the consumers' costs down. This industry remains profitable by lobbying politicians. Recognize, if a person can go to another state to fix the family car for less money, or buy goods for a cheaper price, why then must people stay within the state of residence to purchase a health insurance policy? In some cases, buying health insurance in a neighboring state could save the consumer thirty-five to sixty-five percent on the purchase. Why is buying insurance not the same as buying any other product?

Competition is how we get accessible and cost-contained health insurance. Our legislators should demand this. Through competition, the terms of insurance policies will improve and the American family might finally have a chance to obtain affordable insurance.

I am sure the insurance industry would love to address any further questions you might have. Remember, it is the insurance companies that grant your claims. Therefore, this would probably be a very good place for you to begin asking your many questions as to why costs are so high, and why quality has been so compromised. But be cautious, your insurance company will now be working hand in hand with the government directly, leaving you in a vulnerable position while trying to obtain decent coverage in the face of rising costs and a growing bureaucracy.

CHAPTER 7

LET'S LOOK AT NURSING

When I entered this profession many years ago, I was very proud to be a nurse. Taking care of the sick was and still is a wonderful skill and gift that I feel very fortunate to have.

As nurses, we are patient advocates. We act as a liaison between the patient and the rest of the healthcare system. We strive to meet your needs by providing and maintaining the highest level of care possible. Sometimes, the challenges we face are difficult, and many times nurses can fall short of patient expectations. Nursing is by no means a perfect profession. Because of this finding, this chapter will be addressing *nursing* advocacy rather than *patient* advocacy, and will explain the plight of the hard-working nurse. I hope that this will give to many a more honest and meaningful insight into this profession that *cares* for you. Although you may find these facts somewhat harsh and critical at times, ultimately, it will give to you the opportunity to evaluate, assimilate, and relate to the nursing profession, which has many problems within. To all my colleagues and co-workers, this chapter is dedicated to you.

Despite the many rewards of nursing, I have found myself suppressed by an industry that strangles most of the thoughts and actions of its nurses. It is now a bureaucracy with constant fear of expensive litigation, never-ending documentation, and the ever-growing protocols for almost everything that is done by its nurses. Those mandatory requirements by government and hospital administration not only take time away from the patients, but they have stifled the talents and dreams of its nurses.

Many nurses today are developing the *I-can't-take-it-anymore* burnout. They have become emotionally and physically exhausted from the everyday demands that have been placed on them. In some cases, the profession has disintegrated into backstabbing and lack of compassion, compounded by the frustration of being treated like second-class citizens. These factors have certainly added fuel to the fire when it comes to the well-known shortage of nurses who have become management's servants. The coffee cup for Christmas, the star on your badge, or the chocolate bar given to you for a job well done, does very little to bolster flagging spirits. Not only do nurses work in this multi-tasked, underpaid, understaffed, and stressful environment, but they find themselves in a career where they are mandated to do a great deal for little return. With an average raise of two percent a year, approximately eighty cents more an hour, their salaries do not keep up with the cost of living. The pay scale is separated by only a few dollars between new hires and those who have worked a lifetime in the field.

Favoritism and lack of administrative support have caused many nurses to question whether they want to stay in this profession. With too many people in charge, departments not working together, and the micro managing interfering with true patient care often results in obstacles that are mind-boggling. Nurses who have risen to management roles often seem to have forgotten what it takes to care for patients. Many times, overworked nurses come to feel that this profession has taken them solely to what is known as "the gates of hell".

Today, there are approximately 3.1 million registered nurses, The average age in the profession is forty-five years old. Since many nurses are now nearing retirement, this will only add to the problem of our nursing shortage and experienced nurses.

Certainly, there are nurses who enter this respectable field because they really care, but it has been shown that nurses have not stayed for very long. Many leave this profession within five years because of job dissatisfaction. I have found that if nurses had the time to really take care of their patients as needed, this shortage would not be present.

Recently, I have noticed that with all the new nursing graduates, many experienced, older nurses are being fired or laid off. They are not being terminated in spite of their skill and dedication, but because of it. Of course, new nurses can bring energy and insight into this profession, but to administrators, they are important because they are less expensive, amenable, and somewhat naïve about administrative demands due to their lack of time in this profession. Ignorance is bliss applies to the eagerness and innocence of these new nurses. This is why seniority no longer exists in this profession.

Nurses are perpetual caregivers who can lose themselves somewhere along the way. They can certainly do for others, but often fall short when it comes to taking care of themselves. Often they experience anger from patients, families, doctors, administrators, and continue to say that everything is just fine, even in the most horrific of situations. Often, they favor martyrdom, for their lives are too often manipulated for the sake of twenty-four/seven scheduling. One needs only to look deeper into this profession to realize everything is not as perfect as it seems. At times, it can be very ugly and diseased. Nurses are often looked down upon by administration when they support peers who are in conflicts with them. However, nurses must learn to not only be advocates for others, but also, more importantly, learn to be advocates for themselves. I question when will nursing management ever learn to stand up and protect its nurses, caring for them the way their nurses care for others? Edicts come easily from administrators, while compassion often remains too hard to find.

It amazes me when I hear of people who work in a grocery store or a department store receiving health insurance for life at their time of retirement. One would think that by working in healthcare this would be the least this industry could provide for its nurses.

Some people say nursing is a great job and more times than not I say this is true, but if you think nursing is like this all the time, then one surely must be not aware of all the issues at hand. We need only to enter the emergency room or doctor's office to realize the true reality of the situation. One will quickly become cognizant that quantity now surpasses quality. Nurses are no longer allowed the important time needed to give patients the kind of care they deserve. What today's healthcare provides is less accessible time to patients, nurses, and other medical staff members. While some patients are very well aware of this fact, we know that many are not.

As nurses and as consumers, we must realize that this is an industry where change is necessary. This change needs to be initiated by its nurses and supported by its administrators. If patient care is suffering and the profession of nursing is broken, then it is time to fix it. We do not need to wait until we find our nurses shouting, "Thanks for the memories," as they stampede out the doors of this profession.

Nurses must ask administrators and the other numerous professional nursing groups to re-evaluate their positions on this profession. They must ask them to stop the cutback of nurses, to stop firing good nurses for minor infractions, and stop increasing the demands in the work place. In addition, nurses need to ask administration to stop blaming its staff nurses for everything that goes wrong, when the rules have never even been written. They need to listen to their nurse's insights and input. Administrators need to realize that their nurses do know what is necessary for appropriate and optimal patient care, and that statistics and data are not the only measurable factors when it comes to this profession. They need to start trusting their nurses and stand by them again. They need to treat their nurses as well-trained professionals, because they do not realize the great harm they have done to the morale of their nurses. There needs to be a change of heart and realization that we, as nurses are all equal. Change can come from the administrators above, but it is also necessary many times to come from the knowledgeable staff below. Administrators and management need to realize that our goals are the same: quality in patient care. Yes, nurses need, and want, to take care of the needs of the patients. However, what is of most importance is the need for nurses to learn how to take care of themselves as professionals. As nurses, we are very highly educated individuals who deserve more than what we are receiving, and I am not just talking about money here.

With regards to the nurses who are pursuing a higher education to teach in this profession, it is necessary that administrators and institutions recognize them when it comes to their deserving efforts. Although sometimes administrators do value this pursuit, they seldom compensate them adequately when it comes to this matter. It would be more beneficial for the people in power to acknowledge this reality and compensate these nurses with appropriate financial rewards for their costly and time consuming accomplishments.

When we speak of people in power, we need only to look to the American Nurses Association (ANA) and ask why this professional organization is so weak. Many nurses do not support this organization because the ANA for the most part only supports patient advocacy. It has fallen short when it comes to the needs of providing, protecting and advancing its nurses. This association in its true sense does not place its nurses where they need and ought to be.

We can no longer ignore these issues. The nursing profession must take care of its own. When this profession learns to treat nurses as true professionals, only then, will we be able to change this image from martyrdom and subservience to the educated and valued people that we truly are. This is something nursing has not done for itself, and needs to be done immediately with great care and consideration for all involved.

CHAPTER 8

LET'S LOOK AT DOCTORS

When it comes to doctors, God bless them all. After spending over a third of their lives preparing to take care of the sick, we must never forget the expenses financial, physical, and emotional that they have incurred in the pursuit of this career. As with any profession, there are the good, the bad, and the ugly, and this is exactly what we will discuss. Not only will we look at the many obstacles that present themselves in their delivery of care, but we will also discuss what really constitutes a good doctor.

I remember many years ago when a doctor entered a nurses' station, the staff would quickly rise and give them their seats. When the doctor gave an order, it would be done immediately. No longer does this occur. Now, what is said is, "That's my chair," and the doctor promptly rises. Staff now questions many doctors' orders and quite often gives their own professional opinions on how to care for the patient themselves. Why has this change taken place?

Years ago, a doctor had a sense of autonomy; rarely does this exist any longer. Now the *hierarchy,* as I call it, runs the show. Not only do doctors need to comply with strict guidelines and regulations with reference to administrators of healthcare and government, but their time is predominantly occupied with addressing the multiple forms from insurance companies and appeasing other demanding authorities. They are told by these controlling agencies the what, when, where and to whom they can give this care. These bureaucrats also tell the doctors how to do it their way, or they will not receive their money. This usually involves the greatest amount of paperwork to be done in the quickest possible time. For these reasons, doctors constantly attend to these mandatory orders to protect themselves from the power of these almighty agencies. As you can see, these skilled warriors are also being suppressed and stifled.

The lack of tort reform by government has allowed patients and lawyers to file endless lawsuits with runaway verdicts causing many doctors to question their profession or even leave it. The cost of malpractice insurance has prompted many to avoid high-risk specializations like OB/GYN, and orthopedic surgery. Most doctors order hundreds of millions of dollars worth of diagnostic tests solely for the sake of defensive medicine. The lengths to which doctors must go to protect themselves against lawsuits have forced them to place the care of their patients on a different level than they did years before.

This profession of medicine has most certainly suffered when doctors must constantly bow to the people who continue to shame the foundation upon which this medical profession stands.

People believe doctors are overpaid, but after working with many doctors, I can see that this is not always the situation. Although many doctors may be affluent, many times, some have not yet reached their financial potential. Their expensive educational loans, long hours and after-hours, on-call weekends, and office overhead must never be overlooked. Most certainly, there are doctors who make a pretty penny for a short time of work, but there are many who put endless effort and energy into their work to receive very little. Doctors who primarily work as clinicians, researchers, teachers, missionaries, or work in other areas of this profession are very overlooked and often underpaid. Remember, money is not always the reason why a doctor becomes a doctor.

What constitutes a good doctor? Good doctors

will be good listeners. Their first responsibility is to understand what the patient needs. Not only do they need to be an excellent clinician and diagnostician, but it is a necessity that they have a good bedside manner. Good doctors need to have a good attitude. Since, they often have to work side by side with colleagues, co-workers, and patients, it is important that they remember that *MD* does not always stand for *majestic deity*. Good doctors need to be accountable and responsible. They need to protect themselves with due diligence, but also maintain their instincts and knowledge. This means they must stop doing every test under the sun, when many tests are not needed. A good doctor needs to be an informed educator, teaching their patients to learn how to take care of themselves and eventually become more independent of this explosive and sometimes dysfunctional healthcare system. Good doctors need to be open-minded and know alternative therapies so people can have other more natural ways to heal.

Doctors need to grow a backbone and tell government and every other agency that dictates their methods of care to get off their backs. They need to put those prescriptions pads away more frequently. They need to realize prescriptions are to be used with discretion and consider the enormous

quantities they too often prescribe. They need to
realize when patients are taking more than a few
medications there is a problem. They need to realize
not all cures come in a pill. Good doctors need to
have a heart. They need to stop standing over the
patients and learn how to look eye to eye with the
patients. Doctors are as human as the people they
serve. Finally, good doctors need to remember why
they became doctors. They need to look inside
themselves and be aware of the reasons they took
that Hippocratic Oath. If their personal insights
prove to be no longer truthful, decent, or ethical, for
their patients or themselves, then it is time for them
to go.

Many years ago, I sustained an injury from a car
accident that caused many fractures to the right side
of my face. When I had my initial surgery, some
thirty years ago, my doctors were not only
technically good, but they were ethically sound
people. Five years ago, the prosthesis placed in my
face was found to have disintegrated. Because of
this, I needed to have further reconstructive surgery
to replace it. A coworker told me that there was a
marvelous doctor who did such operations. Thus, I
proceeded to venture into a nightmare that still
haunts me to this day.

After making an appointment with this doctor, I

was told not only did I need this prosthesis replaced, but also a mini-lift would be necessary in order to give symmetry to my face. Although I told him twice that I only wished replacement of the cheekbone, he was adamant that this additional surgery was necessary. Believing this doctor, off I went to surgery. When I woke up, I found the doctor looking over me telling me everything went beautifully. While getting dressed after recovery, I looked into a mirror and was terrified at what I saw. On the left side of my face (the side not affected by the original car accident), I found a gaping hole along the suture line of this "needed" mini lift. On the right side of my face, swelling was extensive and I was unable to pucker my upper lip. In my post-op appointment twenty-four hours later, he said this was to be expected and it was normal for this type of surgery. At this same time, I also questioned why there was a slight protrusion of what seemed to be the prosthesis itself, but I was told once again, that this was not a problem. As the weeks passed, I made another visit to see this doctor. I told him the right side of my face was flat with no signs of cheek definition. To this, he told me that he put the largest prosthesis that he had at the time into the cheek and that was that. When I questioned him about having a second opinion from another doctor for possible consult and revision, he promptly responded, "No one will ever need to fix the work I have done." I could not believe the arrogance of this man. I believed accountability for what was done incorrectly should have been of the utmost importance here, but what I found instead was an inflated ego that took precedence over the patient. (In this case, the patient was me). Eventually, this man did return part of the fees I paid, but he never compensated me for the injury. He kept the insurance payment for the surgical suite and for anesthesia, and the rest...I don't really know where it went. One year later after two neurological consults, I found out that my facial and trigeminal nerve was partially severed by the surgery and that I would have intermittent paralysis and twitching on the right side of my face for the rest of my life. I called this doctor's office to inform him of these findings, and the office manager said that the doctor would not be talking to me and that this case was closed.

One might ask why I could ever have allowed this to occur. Actually in the interim, I tried to obtain a doctor to testify against this man's work, but what I received from consulting doctors was that yes, it was done incorrectly, but they could not testify against him. Why, because they had to work in the same county as this man and therefore it would not be in their best interests to get involved in such a case. I finally did find a doctor out of the county, but the only problem was the $20,000 he wanted to review the previous doctor's findings and just to begin preliminary court proceedings. Being recently widowed and a mother of two, I decided to place my savings and my children ahead of what this self-serving and unaccountable doctor did.

What is the point of all this? First, patients beware; secondly, always know who and what your doctor is all about. Remember, what you are told is not always what is right and true for you. Realize that you can become a victim, if you do not do your homework. Remember, personal integrity does exist, but not in everyone. Believe in your instincts, because, most of the time, they are correct. If you ignore them, you will certainly pay a costly price. It will not only be financial, but physical and emotional as well. Never falter in what you believe is your truth. This is especially important when it comes to your health.

CHAPTER 9

LET'S LOOK AT HOSPITALS

When one sees those shiny floors may I say do not mentally connect
For on its surface and underneath will be things that will infect
Only look to recent findings and one will utterly be surprised
That these hospital acquired infections are most certainly on the rise

The penalties for such infractions and the regulations are very high
So, when it comes to government one better take a big sigh
With hospitals already struggling with their own financial woes
This is just another burden that these institutions must tow

While talking about finances, may I only come to say
That when one chooses to bunk the night one definitely will pay
The costs are high, the accommodations just so
But if one were to choose the Ritz Carlton, I'd say, "Definitely let's go"

For although these hospitals have to charge thousands for those elaborate scans
May one only realize that one has the cost of technology and other issues in their hands
Only look at those $50 pills that are charged so easily
May one realize that these adjustments have been done somewhat sleazily

One knows this is not to punish you, for most everyone needs some pills
For if they did not do this who else would pay those bills?
So for all those who are using and do not wish to pay
May I say, "This is just a small sample of what we need to say"

You have congested the halls, you have abused in an indecent way
For this self-convenience the innocent must pay
Now patient safety and mission statements are of the greatest concern
But institutions, you must look above and ahead and also try to learn

That the quality of care most certainly starts at the top
And what one might be doing may just not be enough
The action needed and the answers sought
Is independent evaluation and reflection that must be taught
To seek this way and do what is right
Hopefully, hospitals will have these correct answers in sight

With this short rhyme about hospitals, we shall now turn to the patients and the staff who work within these facilities. Here, we will learn not only what actually encompasses a good patient and staff relationship, but what is necessary to make these relationships work well when it comes to quality of care.

CHAPTER 10

LET'S LOOK AT PATIENTS/CLIENTS AND STAFF RELATIONSHIPS

When people are sick, whether physically or emotionally, we need to remember: that it will not be the medical staff who will lead the patient into health, nor the patient leading the staff. It will be a mutual relationship during the course of treatment that will take each person involved to a higher level of well being.

When it comes to patient care, the first thing necessary for a mutual relationship is the balance between client and staff. Often, I think of this relationship like a seesaw. The balance relates to the *power* that both parties wish to achieve in the relationship. If this balance of power is not maintained, it can lead to an inability to cooperate with one another. If not correctly utilized this power can and will do harm to the quality of care that both parties want. Not only will patients suffer, but staff and families of patients will also suffer. It is essential for patients and staff to work together harmoniously, otherwise conflicts will arise. The following are examples to explain the importance of this patient-staff relationship.

As we know, nurses share more information with patients than any other healthcare provider group. They are not only involved with the patients, but many times, they are involved with family members and other staff as well. Often, when nurses make a decision of how many family members can be at the bedside of a patient, sometimes, this decision can upset many. In these circumstances, in order to maintain a balance of each ones individual power, what needs to occur is the awareness and acceptance that everyone needs to put the patient's needs first. This is for the sole purpose of quality of care to the patient. When this mutual understanding and relationship takes place, not only are decisions made in a harmonious way, they are made to the benefit of all.

Another example of patient-staff relationships occurs when patients come into a facility for treatment. One of the first things done for the patient is to give them papers concerning their patient rights. Often, this involves their rights to privacy. Sometimes these rights are not upheld. Frequently, medical staff can catch themselves speaking about confidential issues without ever realizing they are in violation of this rule.

At other times, we can see just the opposite when the patient can be the one who is in violation of the rights of the nurse or other staff members. Often, a patient can berate a nurse or other member of the medical team when they are only trying to do their jobs. For example: When drug seekers want their narcotics and don't receive them, they can often become irate if they don't get what they want. Here, what needs to occur is once again a mutual respect for one another. Although, the patient needs to be acknowledged for what they are speaking out for and what they need, they must realize that this care needs to be appropriate for them and done in a manner that shows respect to all. This is known as a medical code of conduct. This is where we connect with one another on a human and ethical level without ever losing respect for both parties' rights. It is not only a necessity to learn this for patient-staff relationships; it is a necessity for mankind to learn also.

When a patient refuses a medication or a treatment, a nurse can become very upset. With this refusal, the nurse will not only have to waste the medication, but other steps will have to be taken as well. Now, the nurse must notify the doctor and the personnel from other specialties on the case, document the occurrence, and probably even get into an elaborate discussion with the patient. This becomes a very complex and lengthened process. Once again, this becomes an issue of power. Often what the medical staff will do is to question why the patient sought help in the first place. Yet, what is necessary here is that the staff learns to open their eyes. They need to realize that patients have the right to choose what is correct for themselves, just as we do every day when we make individual decisions for ourselves. Although clinically, we may believe they should comply with what we feel is right, we should never forget they also have a right to differ with us. It will be in this partnership of understanding, acknowledgement, and balance that we will pave the necessary ground for both to obtain what is right.

When looking at staff-patient relationships, I have many times seen incredible rapport, but at other times I have seen very little. When a patient sees a medical staff member with enthusiasm, great skills, confidence, and joy, they see professionalism. When a staff member has this, they have passion, to which all patients respond. It is in this area that we find knowledge connecting with mutual trust and reciprocation. It is only when people strive for these qualities that they can ever begin to have a sense of balance in their own general lives. Here, this is especially important when it comes to patient/staff relationships. Patients have expectations of what they need. As part of the healthcare team, we need to be aware of these expectations at all times. When it comes to patients, no matter what their mood or temperament, we need to remember to be decent to one another.

As a patient/consumer, one has many rights:

- The right to have considerate and respectful care
- The right to be well-informed about any treatment or procedure performed
- The right to accept or refuse treatments
- The right to confidentiality
- The right to expect the care they receive will be the best it can be

As a patient, one also has responsibilities:

- They are responsible for providing information that is relevant to their care
- The responsibility to ask questions, and to be clear on any instructions given to them
- The responsibility to provide accurate information and to pay for services rendered
- The responsibility of following instructions

to complete their care

- The responsibility to inform healthcare if their safety or dignity has been compromised during their care

When healthcare learns to blend with patients, and patients with staff, we will see excellence in healthcare. It is through this knowledge of whom we are, what we know, and what we believe in that we will eventually come to know what true partnership and power is. If together we were to own this power in this partnership, we then could bring about a different kind of healthcare that would be beneficial to all.

In the following chapter, you will learn how to really get healthy. There are only five steps necessary to obtain this goal. Ultimately, health will be yours, but only if you choose to have it. If you are open-minded, you will find the healthy life you have been looking for. By making correct choices and by making the necessary changes in your lifestyle, you will be able to say that you are no longer a patient, but rather now you are an individual who has found the meaning of an exceptional type of health.

CHAPTER 11

LET'S LOOK AT HEALTH

Health is not just the absence of disease. It is a state of well being. Buddha once said, "The secret of health for both the mind and the body is not to mourn for the past nor to worry about the future, but to live in the present moment wisely and earnestly." With this wisdom, we can now learn how to obtain health in its truest sense. Finally, we can reclaim this life of well-being that we were very much designed and destined to have.

Working many years as a nurse, I have learned that the human body is one of the most magnificent machines ever made. It tells us everything that we need to know. Whether by signs, symptoms, or by pain itself, it talks to us. For this reason alone, we need to have respect and reverence for such a wonderful creation. For many people, they only come to realize this when they have chronic disease, have become gravely ill, or when they are facing death itself.

Previously in the book, we looked into the emotional and physical issues of disease. Now, we shall look at the fundamentals of what the body actually needs in order to overcome most diseases and illnesses. The following steps to health are precise and need to be done in the order presented. Although some of these steps are well known, many are not, so let us begin this journey together.

When we are born, we are given a natural immune system, which provides protection against disease. As we grow, we can make poor decisions that will eventually lead us into illness. When we choose to eat and drink incorrectly, we destroy the natural defense that has been given to us. Thus, we become vulnerable by the choices we make.

When it comes to health, one needs only to remember the saying, "You are what you eat." The importance of these words should never be underestimated. The quality of the food that we consume is of great importance, yet how we assimilate it (take it in and process it) is of even higher significance. Because of this, the first step to health will be the necessity of cleansing our bodies. Before we can ever properly re-energize and nourish ourselves, we need to acknowledge the importance of the process called "detoxification". After this process has been done, the body will finally be ready to take in the essential nutrients necessary to sustain life. For many people, these nutrients have probably been missing in their bodies for many years.

Many people believe cleansing/detoxification can be done with the use of over- the-counter laxatives or enemas, but this is not true. After eating poorly for many years, we need to prepare our bodies by removing the caustic toxins that have accumulated during our lives. Since *these toxins can be a breeding ground for diseases*, we need to eliminate them. To illustrate this point, I ask only that everyone reading this take out a piece of meat, cook it, or leave it uncooked, and keep it out for two to three days. This is the approximate time it takes for your body to completely digest meat.

What you are seeing is what is occurring in your body. It is this meat that is clinging to the linings of your intestines, not to mention other foods that we have consumed. This is why it is essential to do a cleansing of the body at least twice a year. For many, this will be one of the most difficult areas of recovery. When this process is completed, you will find the eventual rewards will be well worth anything you had to experience during the process. Some easy methods for detoxification are as follows:

SENNA LEAVES:

These herbs gently remove waste and purify the colon. It detoxifies the liver and facilitates the absorption of vital nutrients. It has anti-inflammatory effects as well as the ability to boost the immune system. It also aids in beautifying the skin.

WHEY:

This powder prevents internal sluggishness, gas, and purifies the intestinal tract. It not only eliminates constipation and toxins, but it will cleanse the colon and facilitate friendly acidophilus bacteria. This type of bacteria will assist with the absorption of many necessary minerals needed for good bones and teeth. It will also lubricate the intestines, and keep the colon moist.

NATURAL INTESTINAL CLEANSERS:

One very good cleanser is by Dr. Schulze. His intestinal cleanser, *#1 and #2*, is a more expensive way of cleansing the colon, but is much easier because it is just a matter of taking a few capsules daily. One can call this company at 1-800-herb-doc.

FRUIT FLUSHES:

These are very inexpensive and accessible ways to cleanse the body. They can be done over a span of three to ten days according to how toxic or abusive one has been with previous foods. With fruit flushes, it is important to drink lots of good, healthy water (this will be discussed later on in this chapter). Remember, that by eating fruits, one will cleanse their body in one of the most natural ways. If one suffers from hypoglycemia or hyperglycemia, it will be necessary to test your blood sugar regularly throughout this type of cleanse. This diet can be done with any ten of the following fruits: apples, apricots, pears, bananas, blackberries, blueberries, cantaloupe, cherries, grapefruit, grapes, kiwi, mangos, oranges, peaches, pineapples, raspberries, plums, strawberries, tomatoes, and watermelons. A great book written on this topic is *The Fruit Flush* by the author Jay Robb. The book is available at www.JayRobb.com or by calling 1-877-JAY-ROBB. It only costs five dollars and you can lose up to nine pounds a week in a very healthy way.

COLONICS:

When it comes to intestinal cleansing, one can use this very popular procedure. Although sometimes controversial, these treatments are available in almost any city in the world. If done correctly, a colonic cleanses the colon while it also facilitates the removal of dead stool from the intestinal tract. This method will remove wastes that have been present for many years in the colon. After just one of these procedures, one will feel ten years younger, and notice a radiant glow in their face and skin. A colonic is often recommended for the following conditions and lifestyle choices:

- Eating processed foods like white bread, ice cream, donuts, etc.
- Drinking soft drinks, coffee, or excess alcohol
- Coated tongue
- Puffiness under the eyes
- Out-of-control blood sugar
- Moodiness
- Insomnia
- Addiction to junk foods
- Overweight or underweight
- Unclear or confused thinking
- Poor memory
- Bulging abdomen with gas
- Prescription drugs taken on a regular basis
- Smoking
- Drinking less than three quarts of water a day
- Constipation

These are all symptoms that your body is *toxic*,

and it's time to clean out the body and start getting back to good health.

The next step toward health is nutrition. We all know that eating fruits, vegetables, whole grains, and legumes is beneficial to our bodies. By eating raw or living food from the earth, we deny any room for dead food. Toxic foods like refined sugar, meats, and dairy do not belong in our bodies. Being living organisms, we need foods that are *alive*. Remember, nothing replaces Mother Nature as Mother Nature herself. What is the reason for this? *When we eat plant-based foods and foods from the ground, we allow our bodies to enter an alkaline state.* This is what is normal for all people. *It is when we become acidic by eating toxic foods that we find our bodies becoming vulnerable to disease.*

When we consume meat, uric acid is created. This acid decreases assimilation and decreases elimination from our bodies. When we take in dairy products, we see the body increasing its mucous production. In simple words, we see congestion occurring that will ultimately lead to a stagnation of the body systems.

Sugar also causes acid to form. When we consume sugar, we draw out calcium as well as other essential minerals like phosphorous from our bones. It amazes me when people are not eating well, or near death, how their doctors suggest a form of liquid nutritional supplement for them. If one looks at these products, they will find they are loaded with sugar, corn syrup, and maltodextrin. Diets high in sugar, fat and dairy are the ones that cause many of our health problems like gallstones, kidney stones, osteoporosis, and even cancer, to mention but a few. These toxic types of diets ultimately affect the natural balance of our bodies, and this imbalance is one of the main reasons why so many people become ill.

Another aspect of nutrition that is important to acknowledge is our need for essential vitamins and minerals. Each vitamin and mineral meets specific needs of the body. If we have a deficiency in one vitamin, it can interfere with other vitamin and mineral functions. If we have too many vitamins and minerals, this can also be dangerous. The over-consumption of vitamins A, B, C, D and E and minerals, such as calcium, iodine, iron, selenium, and zinc, can lead to problems and should be used with caution. Vitamins and minerals are necessary for good growth and good health. It is always better to receive them through our diets so the danger of excess is minimized.

Essential *enzymes* are also a very important aspect of nutrition. While many people have heard of enzymes, many are not aware of their necessity.

Enzymes are molecules that increase the rate of a chemical reaction. They help break down nutrients, allowing them to be absorbed by our bodies. They are imperative for the digestion of food and valuable in the conversion to, and elimination of, waste. Their most valued asset is that they help cleanse the blood. Remember, the blood is the river of life and it helps dispose of these deadly wastes from our bodies. Enzymes work with and facilitate this function. They restore the body to a steady state. When the immune system is low in enzymes, it will not assist the body in the creation of necessary antibodies to fight infectious diseases. When diseases like multiple sclerosis, rheumatoid arthritis, and lupus bombard our immune systems, they will slow down our bodies. Enzymes help the body respond more efficiently to the toxicity of these diseases. Enzymes have been discovered to have anti-fibrotic effects also. Thus, for all those with thick blood, one may just want to look into these important nutritional supplements. In addition, enzymes are often found to have very few side effects.

When we have decreased enzyme levels, we once again see our bodies more prone to illness. Decreased enzyme levels will leave food poorly digested, which will cause it to ferment and poison the body. Deficiencies of such enzymes can lead to kidney disorders, high blood pressure, diabetes, food allergies, digestive disorders, migraines, anxiety, psoriasis, depression, fatigue, premature aging, and other long-term health problems. For these reasons, we need to realize the choices we make about our diets can and will be one of the leading causes and culprits of disease. It is an absolute necessity to choose our diets and supplements wisely. One also needs to be careful when it comes to over-the-counter vitamins, minerals, and enzymes. Just like anything else, we need to make sure what we take into the body is of the utmost quality.

Another necessity for the body that is of great value and is one of the greatest foods on earth is Blue Green Algae. Not only is this product high in neuropeptides (brain food), but it also has high quality proteins, beta-carotene, B vitamins, and other essential nutrients that can help the body function properly. The quality of this protein is almost identical to the perfect amino acid (protein) profile of the human body, and it even strengthens the immune system. It is not a supplement, but rather it is a whole, organic food. Since we are all organic beings, we need to consume foods that are natural for our bodies. Blue Green Algae is such a unique food with its high quality nutrition that in only a few days one will feel it's true benefits. Often, the results can be felt in as little as an hour. By using Blue Green Algae, one will have a much higher energy level, and will experience greater mental clarity.

Other benefits of this product are better digestion and assimilation of food, decreased depression, fewer or no sweet cravings, weight stabilization, decreased allergic reactions, more respiratory clarity, less inflammation, leveled blood sugar, decreased heart palpitations, easier sleeping at night, fewer muscle cramps, decreased headaches, more relaxed persona, a better attitude, and a calmer disposition. One of the biggest and most impressive findings is with Parkinson's and Alzheimer's disease. In as quick as a few days, incredible improvement in body function is often seen. Remember, while taking this food you need to eat properly. This will mean no further processed or refined foods. This complete balance of vitamins, minerals, enzymes, and nutrients will finally give many what they have been missing: a state of good nutrition and feeling of well-being. Start slowly with one or two capsules or teaspoons, once or twice daily for four days and then gradually increase the amount until you notice its positive effects. Usually, this occurs with 1-2 tablespoons every morning and night. When taking this product, I prefer the liquid form in a little juice, when taking this food. *Consistency in taking this daily is the key.* You can purchase Blue Green Algae at any health food store, find it online at www.E3Live.com, or order by telephone at 1-888-800-7070. Please note, this is not a paid endorsement for this or any other products mentioned in this book. I just need to share with everyone that this is a terrific product that really works. If you are a poor eater, it is essential to take these products to support the body's return to a better state of health.

The next step that is imperative for good health is *hydration/water.* Today, soda, coffee, and energy drinks play a very large part in the American diet. Many people have become too dependent on these liquids for their fast sugar rushes and the stimulatory effects of caffeine. What many fail to realize is how these products can create devastating effects on the heart, kidneys, and other parts of the body. For these reasons alone, we need to look at water as the alternative and ultimate solution for hydration of our bodies.

Since we are organisms that are seventy percent water, it is essential that we replenish our bodies with the correct water necessary to support life. For many years, rainwater was considered the safest source of water, but with pollutants and contaminants in the air, it is no longer healthy for us. So what should an individual do? The answer is to drink distilled water, Many would differ with this opinion, but because water is of such profound importance to our bodies, I will elaborate on this issue.

Many are under the false impression that tap water and even bottled water produced by filtration is pure. This is not true. Tap water is loaded with many pollutants and toxins. Many contaminants make it through filtration and the filters used in this process often become breeding grounds for bacteria. Because of this, filtered water may actually become more contaminated than the water source itself. Contrary to filtration, distilled water is created by heating, and then condensing it into a liquid. It is because of this process that distilled water becomes very close to what we would consider pure.

Many people ask why drinking pure water is important. When we drink impure water, the body must act as a filter, trapping inorganic minerals and other impurities in our bodies. If we allow this build-up to occur, we can cause great harm to our bodies. This includes many diseases, especially those of the liver, kidneys, and intestines. We need to rid ourselves of these inorganic minerals, which the body neither stores nor assimilates. Distilled water is the best water for preventing these wastes from stagnating in our bodies. Since distilled water does not contain inorganic minerals like spring water and well water does, distilled water is a better choice. *Further, distilled water does not leech out the organic minerals from the bones, thus we have an environment that is more conducive to preserving important minerals.*

On the other hand, hard water, such as tap water, is composed of inorganic minerals that clog the arteries and plumbing of our bodies. Some case histories have shown that calcium build-up can cause problems like arthritis and even heart attacks. Calcium, as well as iron deposits, have also been linked to high cholesterol and hardening of the arteries that we see so often. Many people think it is just fat that does this to our arteries, but if you do not keep the natural flow of the blood going to the body and hydrate it properly, one will see difficulties like this occurring. That is why fruit and vegetables are so important because they give you the *organic* minerals and natural complex vitamins that are good for you.

Simply changing hard water to soft water is not purification. Hard water is usually converted to soft water by adding salt (sodium chloride). The body can have difficulties assimilating this added sodium. In many cases, this can affect the body's electrolyte balance. One of the reasons skinny people can have high blood pressure is because of the added salt in soft water. Doctors advise patients on sodium free diets to drink distilled water. When the electrolyte balance in the body is changed, it can sometimes affect your blood pressure.

Pure water will help keep arteries and organs healthier. Hospitals utilize distilled water in their dialysis machines. Yes, that's right...distilled water. This is because the kidneys and dialysis machines cannot maintain themselves if their delicate filter systems are congested with inorganic minerals from other types of water. Distilled water has no strain on the kidneys nor does it usually compromise any organs.

Many people choose not to drink city water because it is filled with chemicals such as fluoride, chloride and other elements. Although these have been said to be beneficial, we must also realize that they are corrosive and poisonous. Chlorine when combined with certain water pollutants has been linked to colon and bladder cancers, with 20,000 new cases reported per year as of 2009. Fluoride has been linked to osteoporosis, high blood pressure, lower IQ, cancer of the bones and problems with gastric damage. Many types of toothpaste contain fluoride. Their packaging even carries a warning to contact poison control if too much is swallowed. This supports the potential toxic effects of fluoride in our water. Fluoride has been linked to thyroid and immune dysfunction, as well as to muscular and skeletal damage.

When we are confronted with these facts, we must ask why there is not more concern about the state of our drinking water. Today, people spend billions a year on bottled water even though the bottles have been linked to cancer. Many serious problems still remain regarding accessing pure water and the safety of its manufacturing.

Here are some interesting tidbits about distilled water: Place a bowl of distilled water and another of any other water in front of your pets and see which one they pick. Give those birds in your backyard some distilled water and see if they return. Wash your hair in distilled water and see how shiny and soft it will become. Lastly, did you know that Secretariat, the fastest racehorse in history, drank only distilled water?

We now know, we can eliminate many of the health problems people are having by drinking distilled water. In this finding, we most certainly have discovered an excellent way to hydrate our bodies. With this being said, may we now raise our glasses with conviction and say, "Let's drink to this," for we have now gained a very important tool for good health.

The next step for better health is increased *oxygen*. As we know, oxygen is more important than water to sustain life. Without oxygen our cells will die, our organs will die and soon we will die. Thus, we can conclude that oxygen is one of the most essential elements for our bodies. When oxygen is depleted or decreased, we learn what the fundamental root cause of most illness is.

As we know many diseases and sicknesses come from anaerobic (unable to live or grow where free oxygen is present) sources. These can be bacteria, viruses, fungi, toxins, and heavy metals. Since these hostile organisms prefer lower levels of oxygen to thrive in, it will be here where we will begin to examine the importance of oxygen and its many therapeutic modalities.

When it comes to oxygen, it is important to first talk about the works of a German scientist, Otto Warburg. This biochemist and medical doctor won the Nobel Prize in 1931, for his research related to the topic of respiratory enzymes and cancer. His ultimate findings showed that cancer could not exist in an oxygen-rich environment. Today, many doctors believe lower levels of oxygen in the tissue cells are a precursor to several diseases. Knowing this, why then do so many people with chronic disease who are treated with oxygen not return to a normal state of health? There are two reasons for this. First, when disease exists, the organs have already been damaged. Secondly, it is the inadequate amounts of oxygen being sent to these organs that usually causes their failure. Because of this, let us then understand more fully a basic concept of oxygen that is relevant to this question.

When we utilize conventional oxygen, it will only help us sustain life. When we use other alternative forms of oxygen like H_2O_2 (peroxide) or O_3 (ozone), we will not only sustain life, but we will cleanse and help heal many diseases. Although this issue of alternative oxygen therapies has been disputed, I believe these alternative methods should be looked at by anyone who is suffering with disease.

The biggest debate over the use of peroxide and ozone therapies usually comes down to its high toxicity when concentrated, which has obscured its many germicidal effects and values. Understand when peroxide and ozone are diluted, and used in proper concentrations, they are not only nontoxic, but they can be uniquely beneficial in healing. We need only look at the increased sales of peroxide that are rising at an average of fifteen percent per year to prove this point. Only look at the FDA, who is constantly postponing the start of ozone and peroxide testing, even though the data has been presented many times over. Here, we need to question why this discouragement of these practices exists. Would it not be devastating to the many healthcare industries concerned, if the availability and cheapness of these products were made known to the public? For this last reason alone, we shall now discuss additional facts related to this type of alternative therapy.

When peroxide comes in contact with anaerobic organisms, they will die. Remember, anaerobic organisms are what cause most disease. When we utilize peroxide on a wound, its bubbling effect is called, *oxidation*. When this occurs, peroxide is killing the molecules inside the shell of these hostile organisms. Not only are the body's cells being boosted with higher levels of oxygen, peroxide is also revitalizing these cells and protecting them. Peroxide is most certainly one of the simplest forms of healing oxygen.

To further explore the beneficial effects of peroxide, we need only to look at the T cells of our bodies. T cells act as scavengers. They patrol the body in the presence of disease. They are the warriors of the body. They seek out pathogens like bacteria, fungi, toxins and metals, and eliminate them by the process of oxidation or perspiration through the skin, colon, lungs and bladder. Did you know that T cells already contain peroxide? It is also found in all fruits and vegetables. Some of the highest concentrations of peroxide can be found in aloe vera, which is one of the greatest healers of the body not only externally, but also internally. High levels of peroxide are also found naturally in breast milk. One of its main functions is to activate and stimulate the immune system. One knows that vitamin C fights infections when given in high doses, but did you know that when given intravenously, it has been found to generate hydrogen peroxide? Lactobacilli found in the colon and vagina produces hydrogen peroxide. This destroys harmful bacteria and viruses, preventing colon disease, vaginitis, bladder infections, and a host of other common ailments. Did you know that before penicillin was ever used, hydrogen peroxide was used for many infections?

This is only a partial list of conditions in which peroxide therapy has been used successfully. You may find diseases that relate to you:

Allergies	Diabetic Retinopathy	Lupus Erythematosis
Altitude Sickness	Digestion problems	Multiple Sclerosis
Alzheimer's	Epstein-Barr Infection	Parasitic Infections
Anemia	Emphysema	Parkinsonism
Asthma	Fungal Infections	Prostatitis
Bacterial Infections	Gingivitis	Rheumatoid Arthritis
Bronchitis	Headaches	Shingles
Cancer	Herpes Simplex	Sinusitis
Candida	Herpes Zoster	Sore Throat
Heart Disease	HIV Infection	Ulcers

As with any treatment, seek the guidance of a provider or doctor experienced in the use of these alternative modalities.

When utilizing peroxide, remember you are detoxifying your body. As with any detoxification, you will feel its effects. When you make changes to your diet, whether good or bad, the cells in your body will react. While the body is removing toxic substances, you may experience headaches, diarrhea, constipation, or rashes. It's possible you'll experience moodiness and even feel a lack of energy intermittently, but this is normal and you'll get through it. Keep reminding yourself that these are the poisons your body has been hiding and they need to be eliminated.

Since I am a nurse and not a doctor, I cannot prescribe, but because I wish to help people with illnesses, I have included formulas you might like to research. Three percent peroxide solution can be purchased at any pharmacy, and although it does not taste as good and as smooth as thirty-five percent peroxide, it can be used.

FORMULA #1:

3% HYDROGEN PEROXIDE PROTOCOL FORMULA

One part of 3% peroxide added to 5 parts distilled water will make a .5% solution of hydrogen peroxide. Using a gallon of distilled water, remove 20 fluid ounces of water. Replace the 20 ounces with 3% peroxide to yield the proper .5% solution. Refrigeration is not necessary. Drink only on an empty stomach since the purpose is to purify the body. Ingest formula one hour before eating or three hours after eating. In the morning and before bed are the usual times for consumption.

1 oz. the first day
2 oz. the second day
3 oz. the third day
4 oz. the fourth day
5 oz. the fifth day
Then Try
5 oz. 3 times per day for 7 days
5 oz. 2 times per day for 7 days
5 oz. one time per day for 7 days
5 oz. once every other day for 7 days
5 oz. once every third day for 7 days
5 oz. once every fourth day for 7 days

When peroxide kills organisms too quickly, it can make you feel uncomfortable. If this happens, back off for a day or two and allow the body to adjust and purify on a comfortable level. You may want to stay on this lower level until the desired results are attained. If your condition is severe, stay on five ounces of the .5% solution twice a day for as long as it deems necessary. The body is cleansing itself and the most important thing is to be at rest and let the body do what it needs to do. Give it as much time as possible to do its job. Eat light foods that are easy to digest: fruits, vegetables, and plenty of distilled water.

FORMULA #2:

OXGENATION PROTOCOL FOR 35% H_2O_2

(This can be purchased online under Oxyplus by Donsbauch.)

Day 1 - 3 drops, 3 times per day
Day 2 - 4 drops, 3 times per day
Day 3 - 5 drops, 3 times per day
Day 4 - 6 drops, 3 times per day
Day 5 - 7 drops, 3 times per day
Day 6 - 8 drops, 3 times per day
Day 7 - 9 drops, 3 times per day

Day 8 - 10 drops, 3 times per day
Day 9 - 12 drops, 3 times per day
Day 10 - 14 drops, 3 times per day
Day 11 - 16 drops, 3 times per day
Day 12 - 18 drops, 3 times per day
Day 13 - 20 drops, 3 times per day
Day 14 - 22 drops, 3 times per day
Day 15 - 24 drops, 3 times per day
Day 16 - 25 drops, 3 times per day equally, up to 75 drops total per day.

Remember, always on an empty stomach, meaning one hour before meals or 3 hours after.

Note: Each day the dose increases by 1 drop, taken 3 times per day except on day 9 when it increases to 2 drops, 3 times per day. If discomfort or nausea develops at any level, stay at that level until discomfort diminishes or simply skip a day to allow the body to acclimate and detox to the new level.

If three times per day is inconvenient, then condense the formula into only two times per day. Suggested mixture is with five ounces of distilled water. Avoid vitamin and mineral supplements unless they are whole food like: alfalfa, kelp, green powders, natural food, etc. Do not mix peroxide in fresh carrot juice, blended bananas, carbonated drinks or alcoholic drinks. The enzyme liberated in carrot juice and bananas destroys the peroxide oxygen molecules. Seventy-five to eighty drops a day of thirty-five percent peroxide will eliminate most harmful bacteria, viruses, fungi, toxins, poisons and heavy metals across the board from most health problems and diseases.

An additional way to utilize peroxide is by purchasing five large bottles of peroxide and pouring them into a tub of hot water. Submerge yourself for thirty-five to forty-five minutes, two or three times per week. Although, this is not as effective as an oral peroxide treatment, your skin will assimilate it and the effects will be close to that of oral consumption.

Another topic of importance is Ozone (O_3). This is a form of oxygen often related to the phrase *pure, fresh air.* To many, it is known as nature's natural purifier and healer. The ozone layer in the atmosphere helps protect us from damaging ultraviolet rays. That is what ozone does, it protect us. It also kills bacteria and viruses on contact. Ozone is simply a high-powered form of oxygen. Ozone has the ability to address many of life's concerns when it comes to disease. It strengthens weakened immune systems and resolves lack of oxygen issues. Ozone (O_3) can perform when at times oxygen (O_2) cannot. The white blood cells of our bodies use ozone to destroy foreign bodies and fight illnesses. Ozone decomposes urea in renal failure. Ozone increases energy production in the cells of the body. This energy is used to protect cells from disease. Proper levels of energy production in cells are essential for a person to maintain and reclaim their health.

When people have chronic disease, they usually have a lower level of oxygen in their blood. It is important to your overall general health that oxygen levels remain within normal limits, but when you are sick, these levels need to be much higher. Since ozone activates enzymes that attack free radicals and neutralize them, we can see by this process that ozone is a very powerful oxidizing agent. It is far stronger than oxygen. It is because of these effects that ozone can assist the body to regain balance and maintain health. Please note: Ozone and peroxide do virtually the same thing, because peroxide is formed when ozone comes in contact with moisture or water.

Ozone therapy is one of the most powerful and natural treatments known in alternative health. Today, many people utilize ozone therapy in Europe, the United States, and other countries. However, there are still many people who remain unaware of its use and benefits. Other utilizations of ozone are by insufflation, steam, ozone-generated machines, and intravenous use. The latter is most useful in chronic diseases of the lung.

In this ever increasingly toxic world, never discount ozone or peroxide therapies simply because you don't understand or know about them. Seek out more information regarding these approaches; they might just save your life and give you the health you have been wishing for and deserve.

The final step in health is *exercise*, which develops the mind as well as the body. It increases oxygen to the body, which will ultimately give us better health. By exercising, we can decrease the risks of heart disease, osteoporosis, breast cancer, and many other diseases. Although people are aware of some of the benefits of regular activity, the list of positive effects is long:

Exercise can:
- Improve digestion
- Enhance quality of sleep
- Add a sparkle and radiance to the complexion
- Improve body shape
- Tone and firm muscles
- Provide more muscle definition
- Enable permanent weight loss,

- Make you limber
- Improve endurance
- Burn extra calories
- Improve circulation and help reduce blood pressure
- Increase lean muscle tissue in the body
- Improve appetite for healthy foods
- Alleviate menstrual cramps
- Increase metabolic rate
- Enhance coordination and balance
- Improve posture
- Ease and help eliminate back problems and pain
- Make the body use calories more efficiently
- Lower resting heart rate
- Increase muscle size through an increase in muscle fibers
- Improve body composition
- Improve bone density
- Decrease fat tissue more easily
- Make the body more agile
- Is the greatest body tune up
- Reduce joint discomfort
- Improve athletic performance
- Enrich sexuality

- Add years to your life
- Increase your range of motion
- Enhance the immune system
- Improve glycogen storage
- Enable the body to utilize energy more efficiently
- Increase enzymes in the body which burn fat
- Enhance oxygen transport throughout the body
- Improve liver functioning
- Increase speed of muscle contraction and reaction time
- Enhance feedback through the nervous system
- Strengthen the heart
- Improve blood flow (very important)
- Help to alleviate varicose veins
- Increase maximum cardiac output
- Increase contractibility of the heart's ventricles
- Improve contractile function of the whole heart
- Make calcium transport in the heart and body more efficient

Even with all these benefits of exercise, it will still be very hard for some people to do. For many, it will take an enormous, concerted effort. One way to reduce this effort is to find something you enjoy doing. If you like to run, then run. If you like to swim, then swim. If you like to dance, then put on those dancing shoes. Whatever activity you choose, if you love it and enjoy it, so will your body. When exercise is fun, it will not only increase your overall stamina, it will also enhance the necessities of what this body and mind were meant to have.

In these days when life's pressures can take their toll, never underestimate where exercise can take you. Not only will it give you a higher level of positive change and direction, it will give you a higher level of preservation and restoration. In truth, it will give you a stronger self-esteem, self-worth, and the presence of a greater self-love. When we learn to finally take responsibility for the lives we live, we will then know what health is all about.

CHAPTER 12

LET'S LOOK AT SOLUTIONS

When we learn to educate instead of medicate, we will finally be on the road to recovery. When we find permanent solutions rather than temporary fixes, we will have actual cures. When we see government no longer granting themselves amnesty from their wrongs, only then will we see justice being done. When we see insurance and pharmaceutical companies finally confessing their misgivings, only then will we no longer need to buy into their ways. When we learn to recognize our bodies as being self-sufficient, only then can we realize the possibility of true change and hope. When people learn to create these necessary changes within themselves, then and only then, will they be taking the medicine so many people find difficult to swallow. When we see people being accountable and responsible for all these new learned findings, only then will we see true health care reform.

As human beings with intellects, we know right from wrong. As we live our daily lives, we need to learn to make better decisions. By making poor choices, we must understand that we will be the ones who will pay the price. By learning from the past and examining the present, we will progress toward a healthier future. *Diaries of a Mad Nurse* was written from practical experiences; never on assumptions. It was written from personal observations and with thoughtful concern. These concerns are not only for the sake of healthcare, but are for the sake of mankind itself.

Today, many people have lost themselves somewhere along the way. They have forgotten what we call virtues and morals. Whether it be lack of money or the love of money, it continues to dictate even when we see the many evils it can create. While abuses continue and people remain unaware of certain situations, we must remember that we, too, are the responsible ones who need to help correct these individual problems.

As we learn to question how we treat ourselves, how to be honest with ourselves and how to treat ourselves differently, we must also learn to be honest with and treat others differently. We need to find out who we truly are. This takes time. Yet, who can ever be more important than yourself?

As humans, we need to seek out and protect our health and our rights. We need to have personal accountability. We need to be active and involved with life, and to choose a life built upon good health and well-being. As we approach this new way of living, we must find the courage and strength to make the necessary changes, with thoughtful wisdom and prudence. When we learn to take in this new kind of knowledge and apply it to ourselves, only then will we have obtained *a higher quality of self-care*.

Truly, this is what health is all about.

SOURCES

"10,000 Baby Boomers Retire." *Daily Number: Baby Boomers Retire.* N. p., n. d. Web. 16 Dec. 2012.

"Average Age of Nurses Increase." N .p., Oct.-Nov. 2009. Web.

Biddle, Sam. "The IN VIVO Blog: July 2007." *The IN VIVO Blog: July 2007.* N. p., n. d. Web. 16 Dec. 2012.

"Can Oxygen Cure Cancer?" N. p., n. d. Web.

"Chlorine, Cancer and Heart Disease." *Chlorine, Cancer and Heart Disease.* N. p., n. d. Web. 16 Dec. 2012.

Christie, Les. "September 13, 2011." *CNN Money.* CNN. N. d. Television.

"CNN's Most Profitable US Companies- 08 By Web Inouye [121 More Lists]." *Ranker.* N. p., n. d. Web. 16 Dec. 2012.

"Employment Situation Summary." *U.S. Bureau of Labor Statistics.* U.S. Bureau of Labor Statistics, 18 Jan. 2013. Web. 16 Dec. 2012.

Goodman, MA, Brenda. "Study: Overuse of Implanted Cardiac Defibrillators." *WebMD.* WebMD, nod. Web. 16 Dec. 2012.

"Health Insurance Industry Profits Surge Again." N. p., n. d. Web.

"Health Insurer Profits Jumped 250% in Last Decade." *DailyFinance.com*. Nap., nod. Web. 16 Dec. 2012.

"How Many People Die of Heart Disease?" N. p., n. d. Web.

Jacobson, Louis. "'Illegal Alien Facts' vs. the Truth-O-Meter." *PolitiFact*. N .p., n. d. Web. 16 Dec. 2012.

Kemble, Tracy, per. *The Right Living Program*. Tracy Kemble. N. d. CD.

"Last Year's Health Care Bill Equaled 2.27 Trillion." N. p., n. d. Web.

"Medical Errors Still Claiming Lives." N. p., n. d. Web.

"Medical Errors Still Claiming Many Lives." N. p., n .d. Web.

Meredith, Peter. "The Truth About Drug Companies." *Mother Jones*. N. p., n. d. Web. 16 Dec. 2012.

"NanomedicineCenter.com." *NanomedicineCentercom RSS*. N. p., n. d. Web. 16 Dec. 2012.

"National Diabetes Information Clearinghouse (NDIC)." *National Diabetes Statistics, 2011*. N. p., n. d.

Web. 16 Dec. 2012.

Nugent, Helen. "Care Home Worker Jailed." *The Guardian*. Guardian News and Media, July-Aug. 2012. Web. 16 Dec. 2012.

"Obesity Rates Among All Children in the U.S." *Centers for Disease Control and Prevention*. Centers for Disease Control and Prevention, 06 Nov. 2012. Web. 16 Dec. 2012.

Oller, Travis. "Many Illegal Immigrants Pay up at Tax Time - USATODAY.com." *Many Illegal Immigrants Pay up at Tax Time - USATODAY.com*. N. p., n. d. Web. 16 Dec. 2012.

"Release RD Legal Funding Offers." (n. d.): n. pg . Web.

Rubenstein, Edwin. "The Social Contract Press - a Quarterly Journal on Population Environment Public Issues International Migration Immigration Language and Assimilation." *The Social Contract Press - a Quarterly Journal on Population Environment Public Issues International Migration Immigration Language and Assimilation*. N. p., n. d. Web. 16 Dec. 2012.

Savage, Michael. "Illegal Alien To The Â U.S." *Arizona Resistance*. N. p., n. d. Web. 16 Dec. 2012.

Schnots, Wilhelm. "Implementation Strategies for Emergency Medical Services Within Stroke Systems of Care." *Implementation Strategies for Emergency Medical Services Within Stroke Systems of Care*. N. p., n. d. Web. 16 Dec. 2012.

Smith, Lamur, US Rep. "U.S. Rep. Says Immigrants Hold 8 Million Jobs." *PolitiFact Texas*. N. p., n. d. Web. 16 Dec. 2012.

Staton, Tracy. "Top 17 Paychecks in Big Pharma." *Fierce Pharma*. N .p., n. d. Web. 16 Dec. 2012.

"Study: Immigrants Pay Tax Share." *Washington Post*. The Washington Post, 05 June 2006. Web. 16 Dec. 2012.

Tampkins, Theresa. "Medical Bills Prompt More than 60 Percent of U.S. Bankruptcies." *CNN*. N.p., 05 June 2009. Web. 16 Dec. 2012.

"Tobacco Use." *Centers for Disease Control and Prevention*. Centers for Disease Control and Prevention, 16 Nov. 2012. Web. 16 Dec. 2012.

"The Truth About Nursing." *The Truth About Nursing*. N. p., n. d. Web. 16 Dec. 2012.

WebMD. WebMD, 10 Feb. 2010. Web. 16 Dec. 2012.

"Welcome to HIPAA 101." *HIPAA Compliance: Regulations, Standards, Certification, Training*. N. p., n. d. Web. 16 Dec. 2012.

Wooldridge, F. "Anchor Babies Away: Enormous Cost of Jackpot Babies to Taxpayers." *Examiner.com.* N. p., n. d. Web. 16 Dec. 2012.

Wooldridge, F. "Frosty Wooldridge -- CONNECTING THE DOTS." *Frosty Wooldridge -- CONNECTING THE DOTS.* N. p., n. d. Web. 16 Dec. 2012.

Writer, Contributing. "What Is the Etiology of Hypertension?" *E How.* Demand Media, 08 July 2009. Web. 16 Dec. 2012.

"YourHealthByDesign.com." *YourHealthByDesign.com.* N. p., n. d. Web. 16 Dec. 2012.

DIARIES OF A MAD NURSE